Best wishes
to your 9th anniversary
Wayland & Roni

EMANUEL

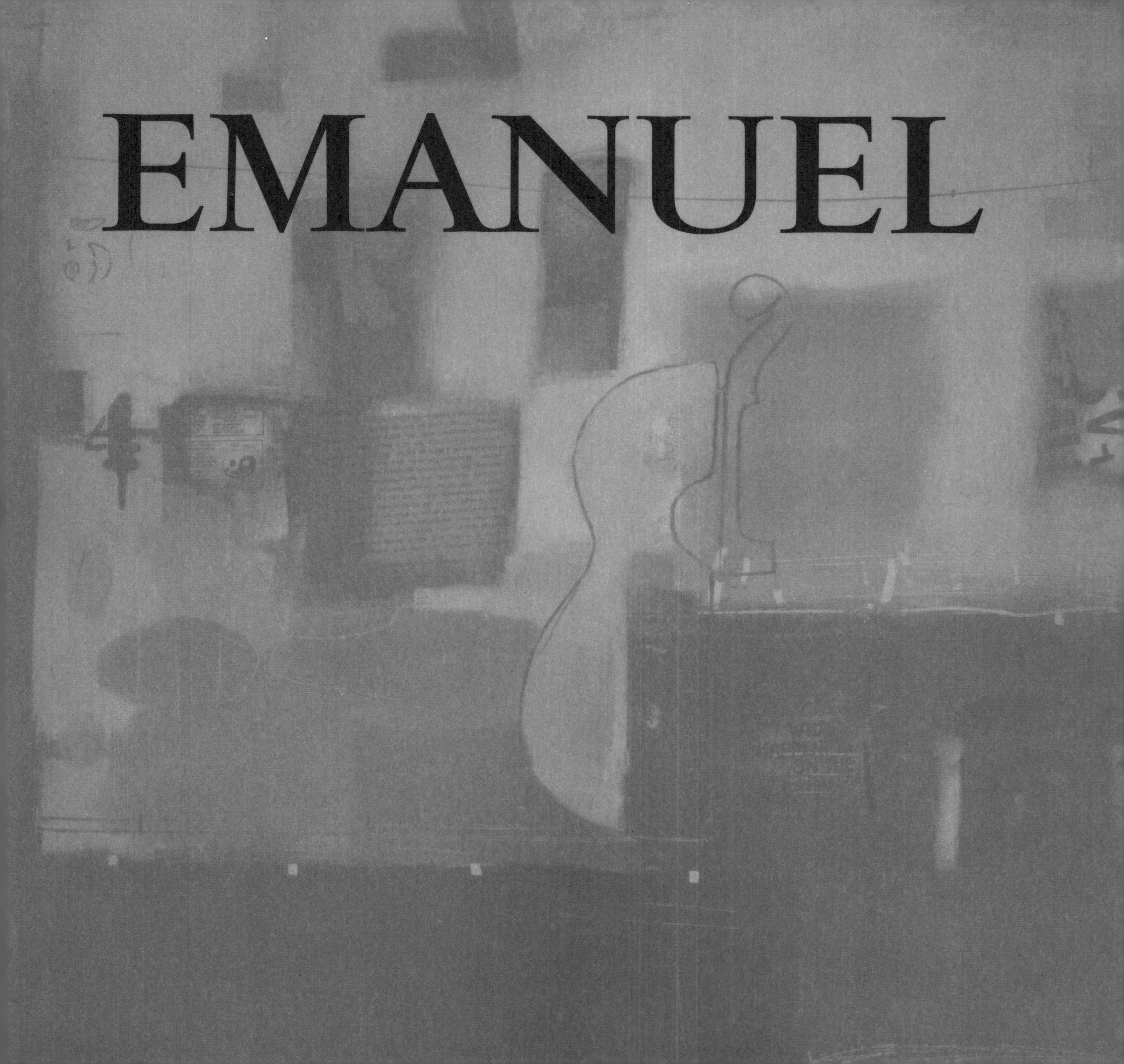

VIGIL OF A WINTER'S MOON

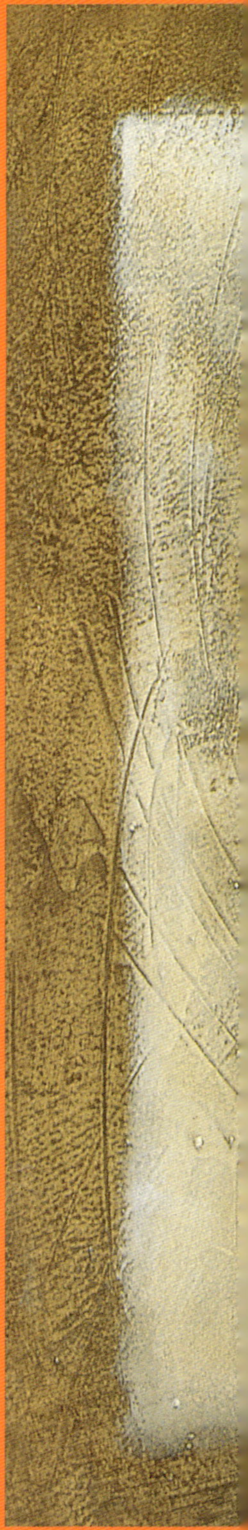

Text by Abbas Daneshvari, Ph.D.

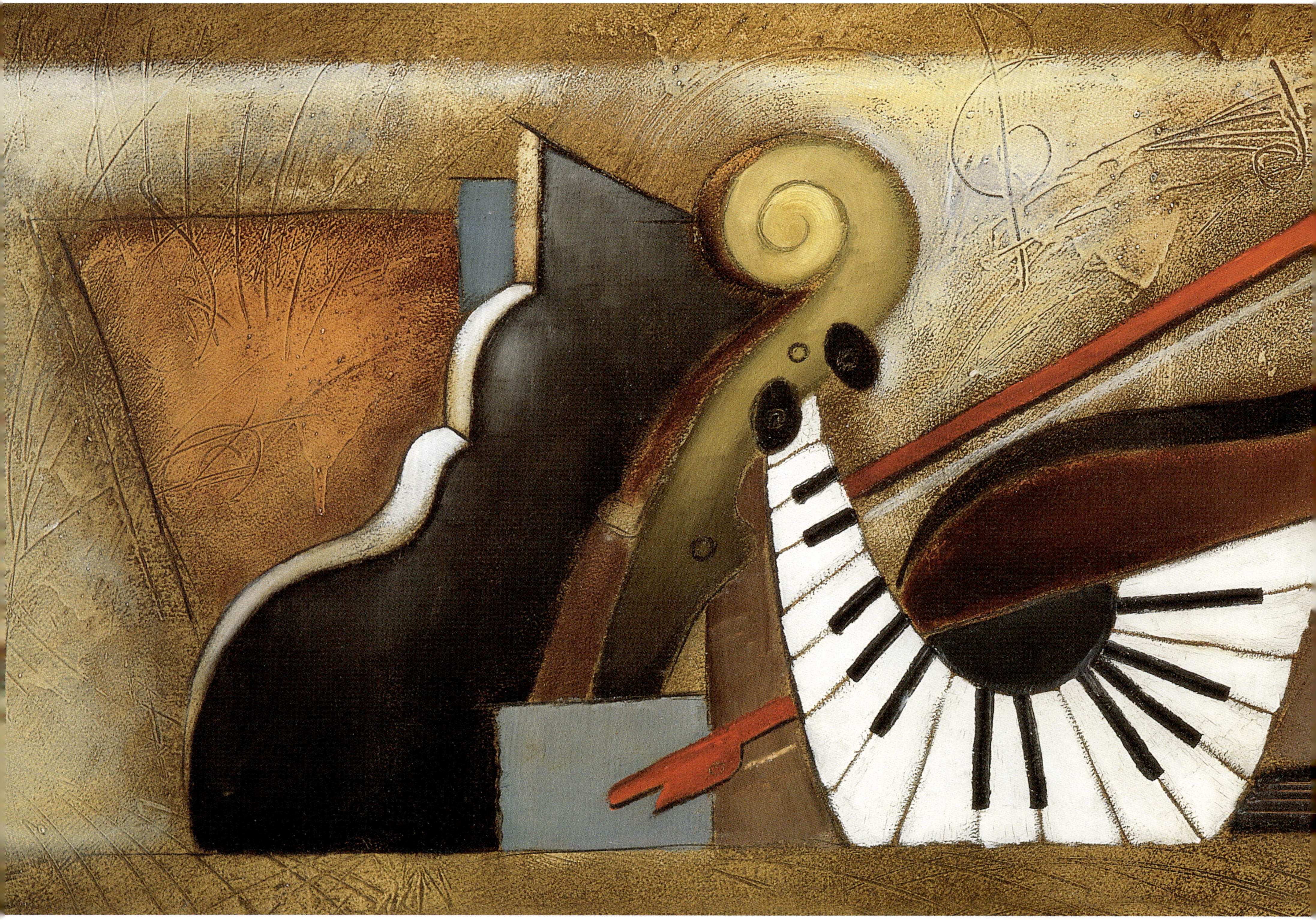

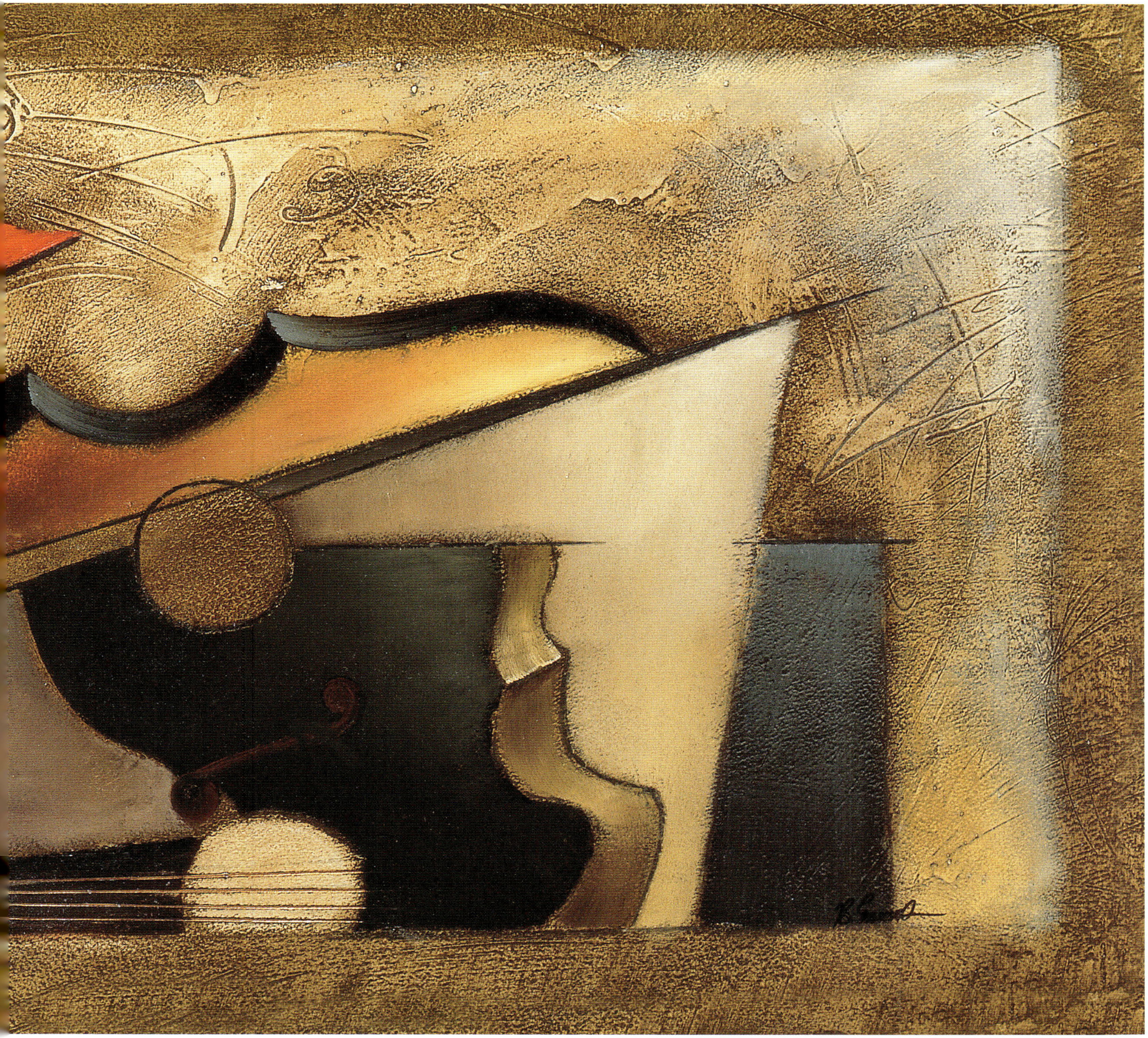

Orchestration X

Mixed Media on Paper 54"x19"

I am pleased and grateful that a selection of my paintings rests within the pages of this book ∾ It is my deepest pleasure to thank all those who have made this publication possible ∾ Above all, I am grateful to Deljou Art Group for being a supportive and caring promoter of my art ∾ They have embraced and given flight to my vision ∾ I also wish to thank Professor Abbas Daneshvari who graciously contributed the text for this publication ∾

Emanuel

It is with pride and immeasurable pleasure that Deljou Art Group, in its pursuit of excellence in the contemporary fine arts, presents this book on the paintings of Emanuel ~ It should, however, be known that this selected compilation of Emanuel's work represents only a fraction of his oeuvres and should be considered an invitation to explore the vision and talent of this young and emerging artist ~

Deljou Art Group

"When I paint I

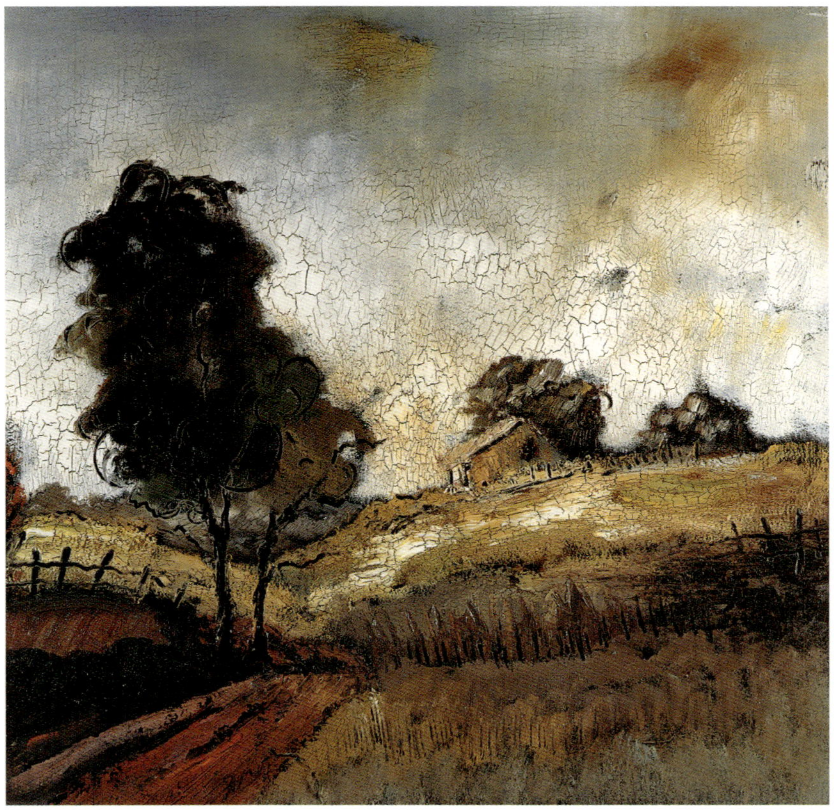

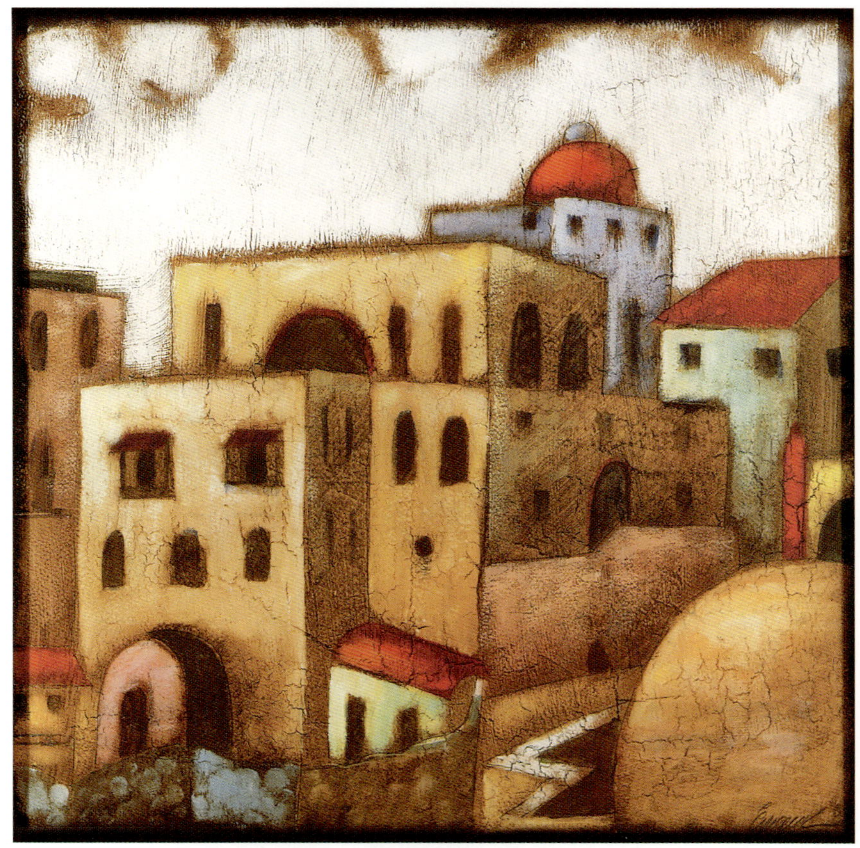

Hallycon Series
Hallycon IV

Casa Series
Casa IX

Mixed Media on Paper 20"x20"

am a song…I am part of a

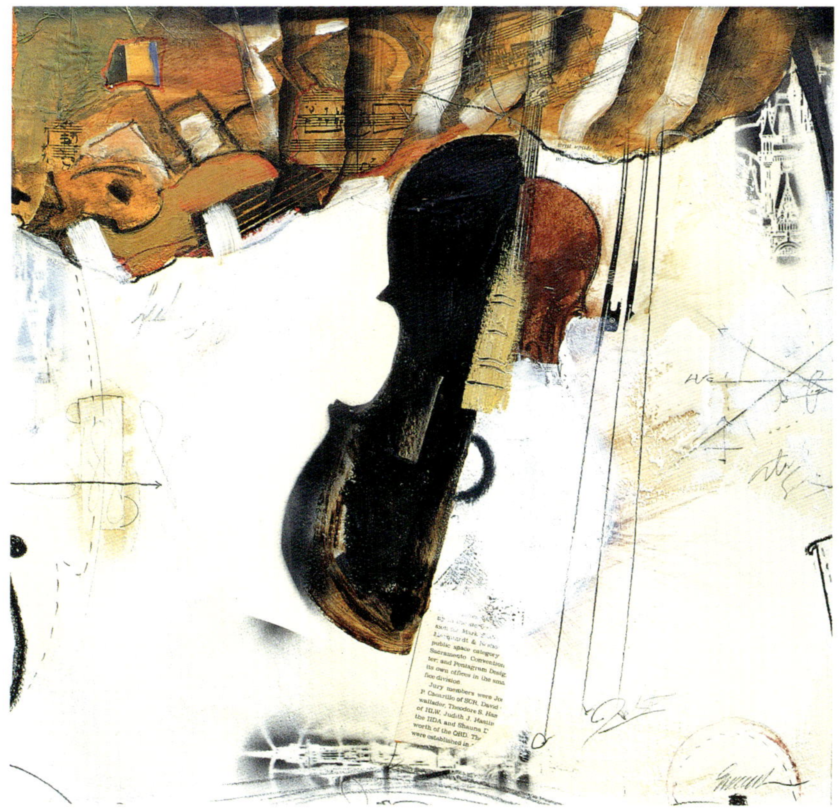

Ledger Line Series
Ledger Line VII

Mixed Media on Paper 20"x20"

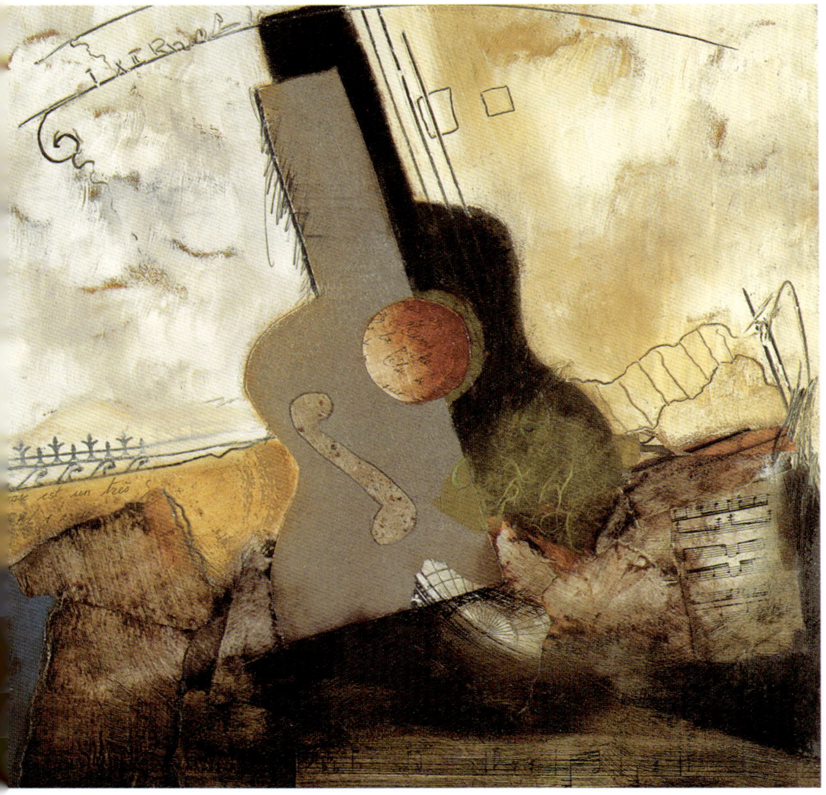

Concerto Series
Concerto I

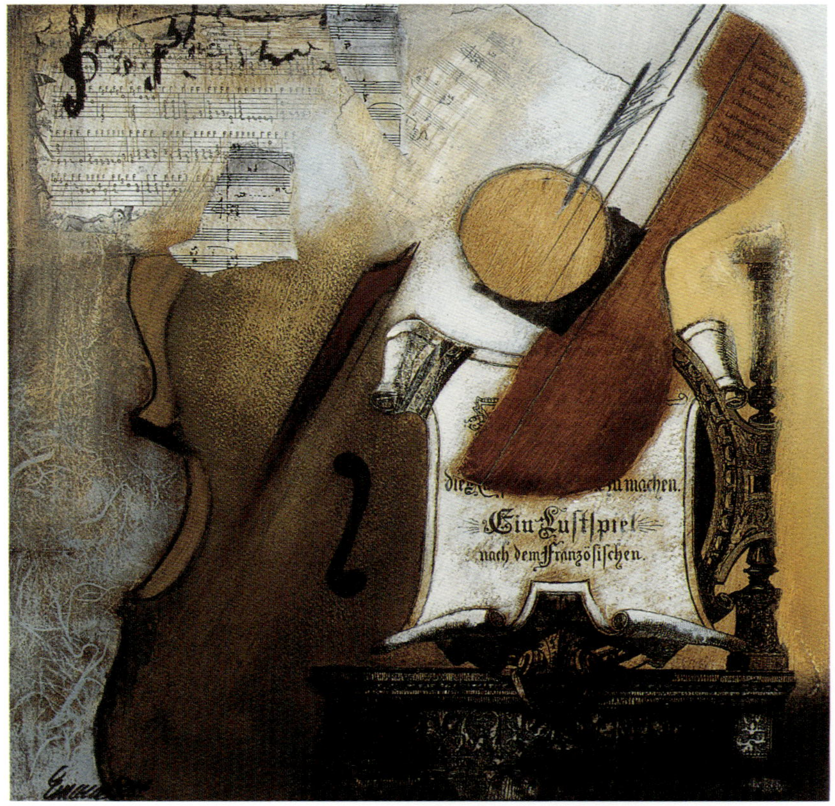

Melodium Series
Melodium VIII

rhythmic flow thrown into

Mixed Media on Paper 20"x20"

Emar

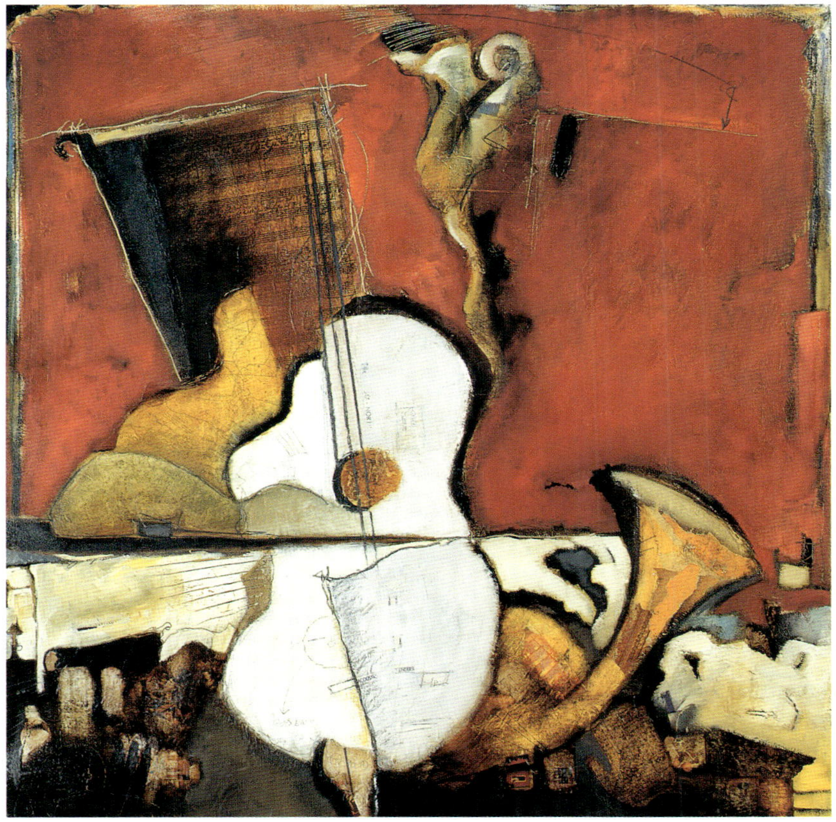

the river of **time.**"

Melodium Series
Red Rondo I

Mixed Media on Canvas 48"x48"

nuel

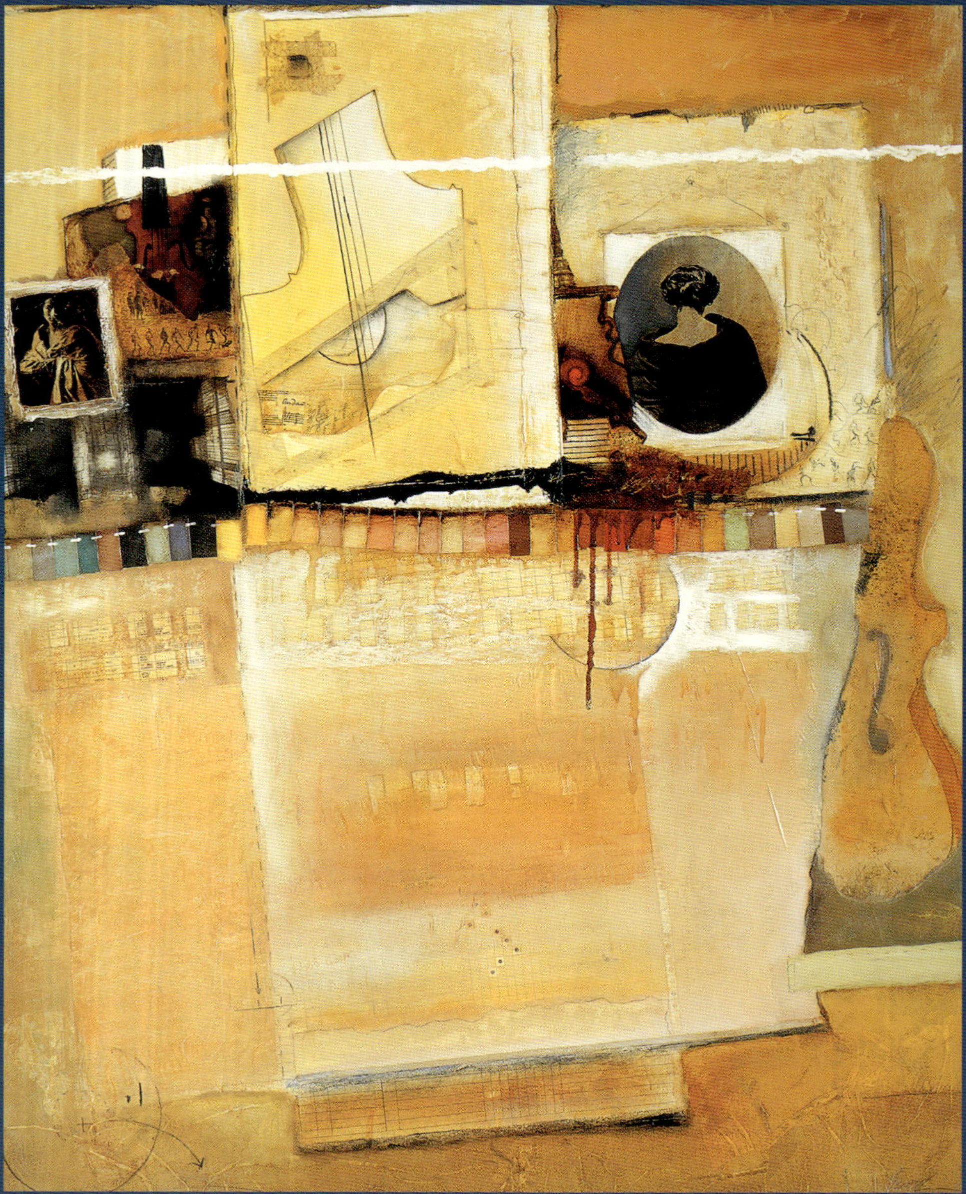

Passages Series
Passage

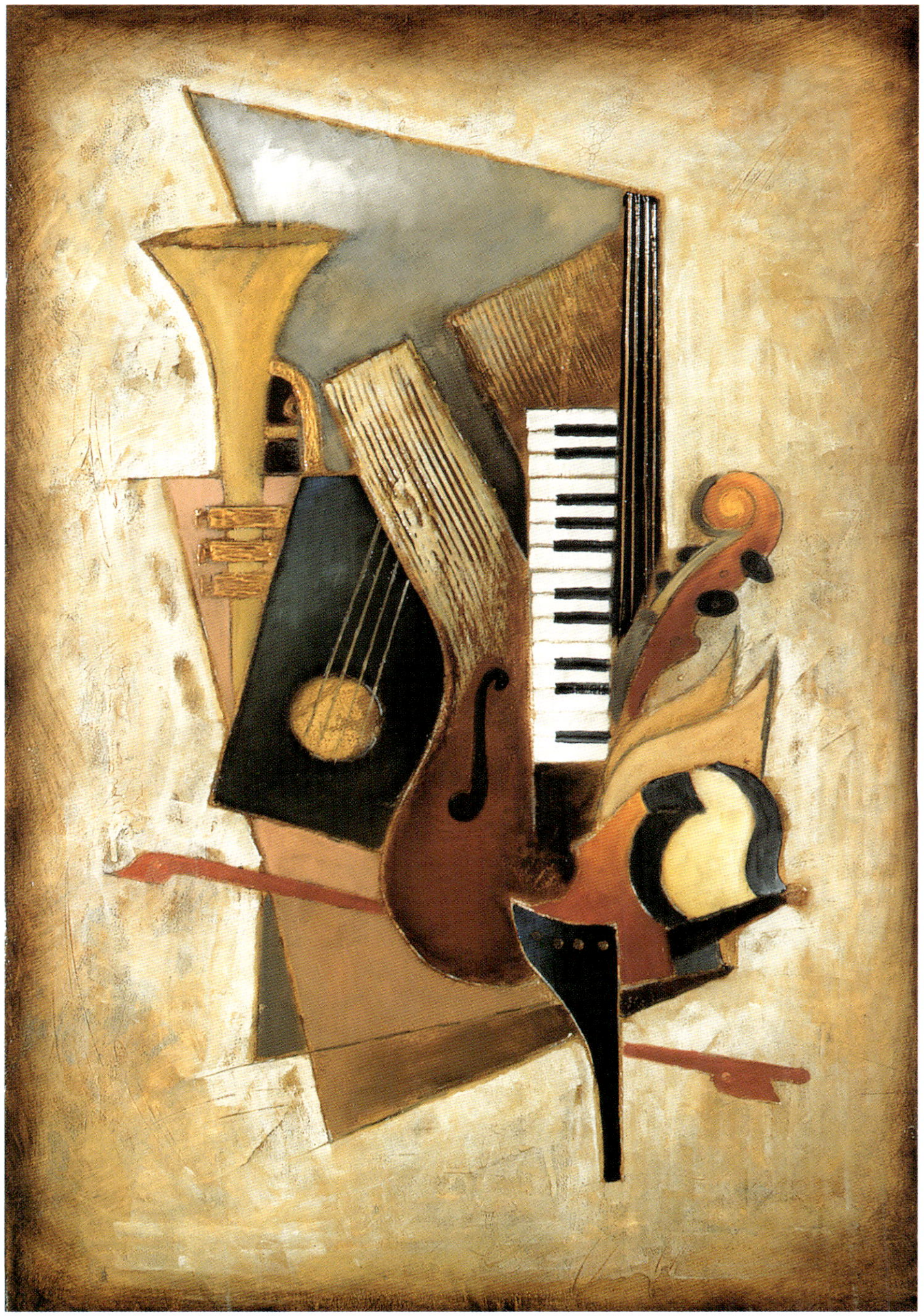

Orchestration Series
Orchestration VII

Mixed Media on Canvas 40"x54"

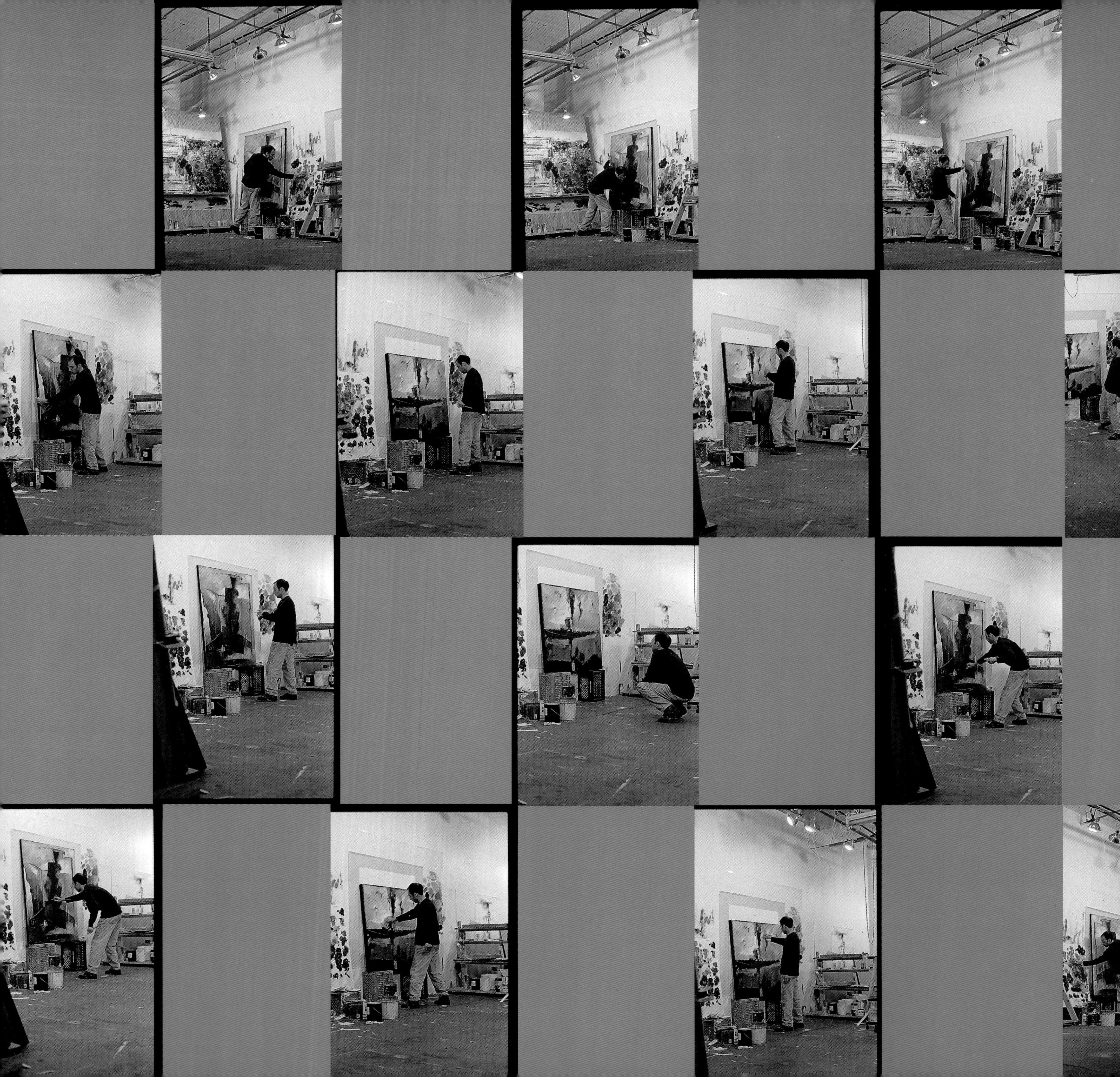

Emanuel was born in Shiraz, Iran. It is serendipitous that this deeply talented and devoted painter should have been born and raised in the heart of Iran's cultural and artistic civilization. The confluence of his native experiences with his American intellectual and artistic journey, bolstered by his education at Georgia State University and the Atlanta College of Art, has sensitized and predisposed him to the vibrations that express the essence of both the western and eastern experiences. In fact, like the Polish-born writer Joseph Conrad, who became an eloquent and original voice for English literature, Emanuel's art is distinguished by its significant stand at a delicate juncture of western art history, reflecting not only its past but also its present concerns and aspirations.

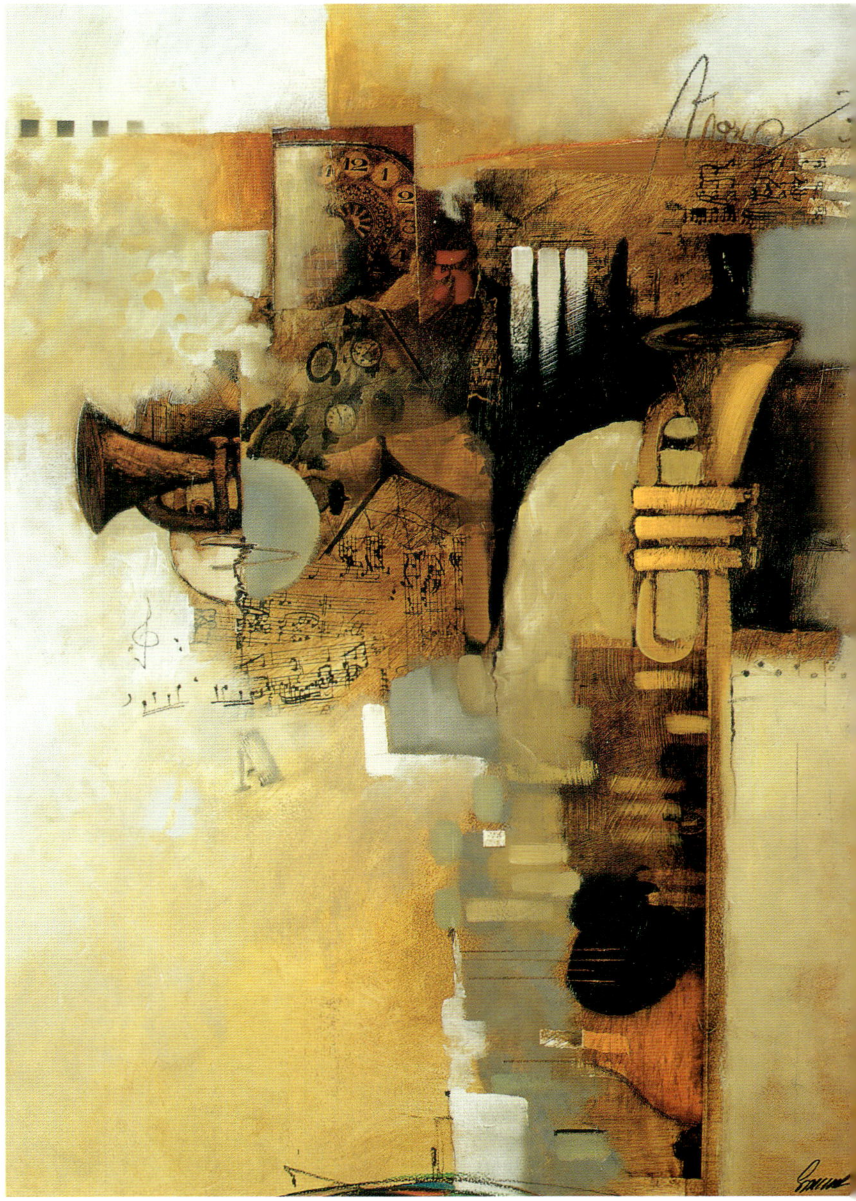

Investigation Poetica I

Mixed Media on Canvas 24"x34"

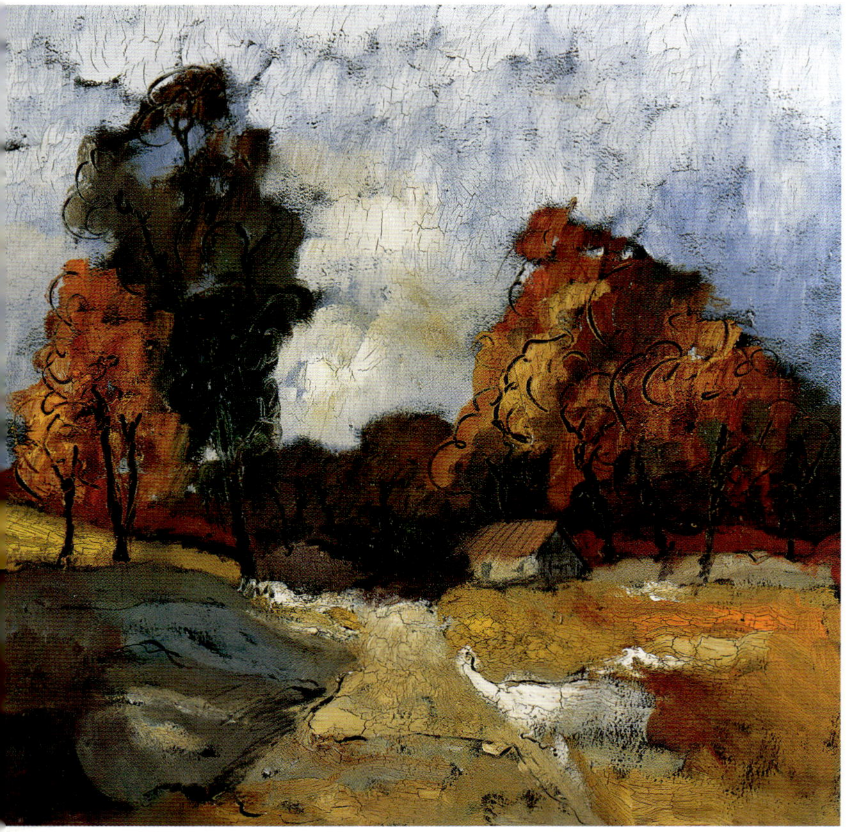

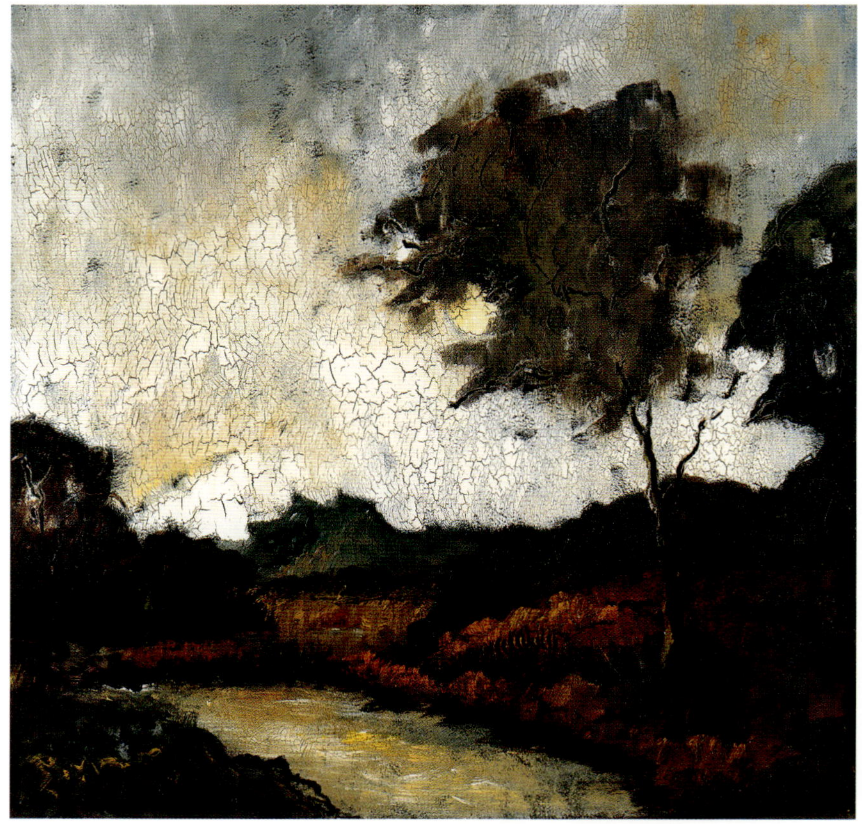

Mixed Media on Paper 20"x20"

Hallycon V

Hallycon VII

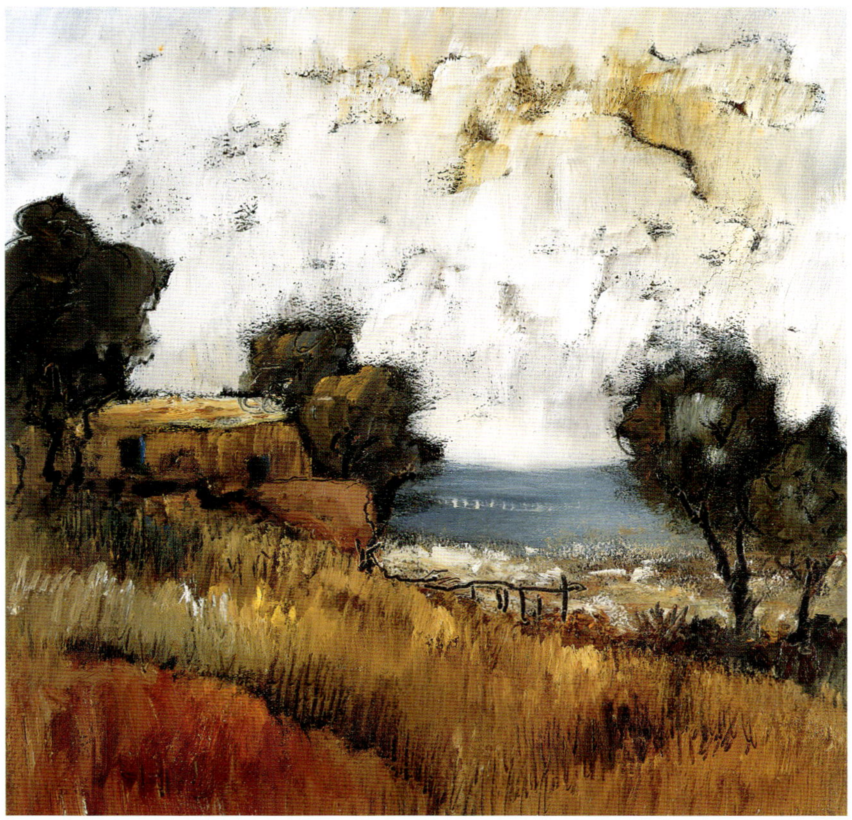

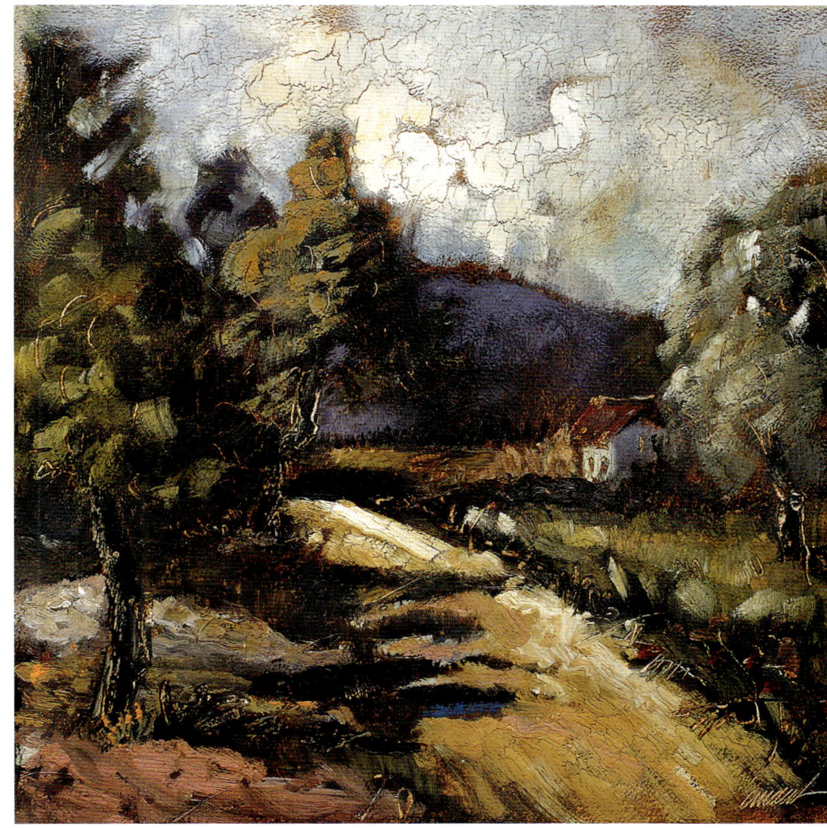

Hallycon VIII

Hallycon X

Mixed Media on Paper 20"x20"

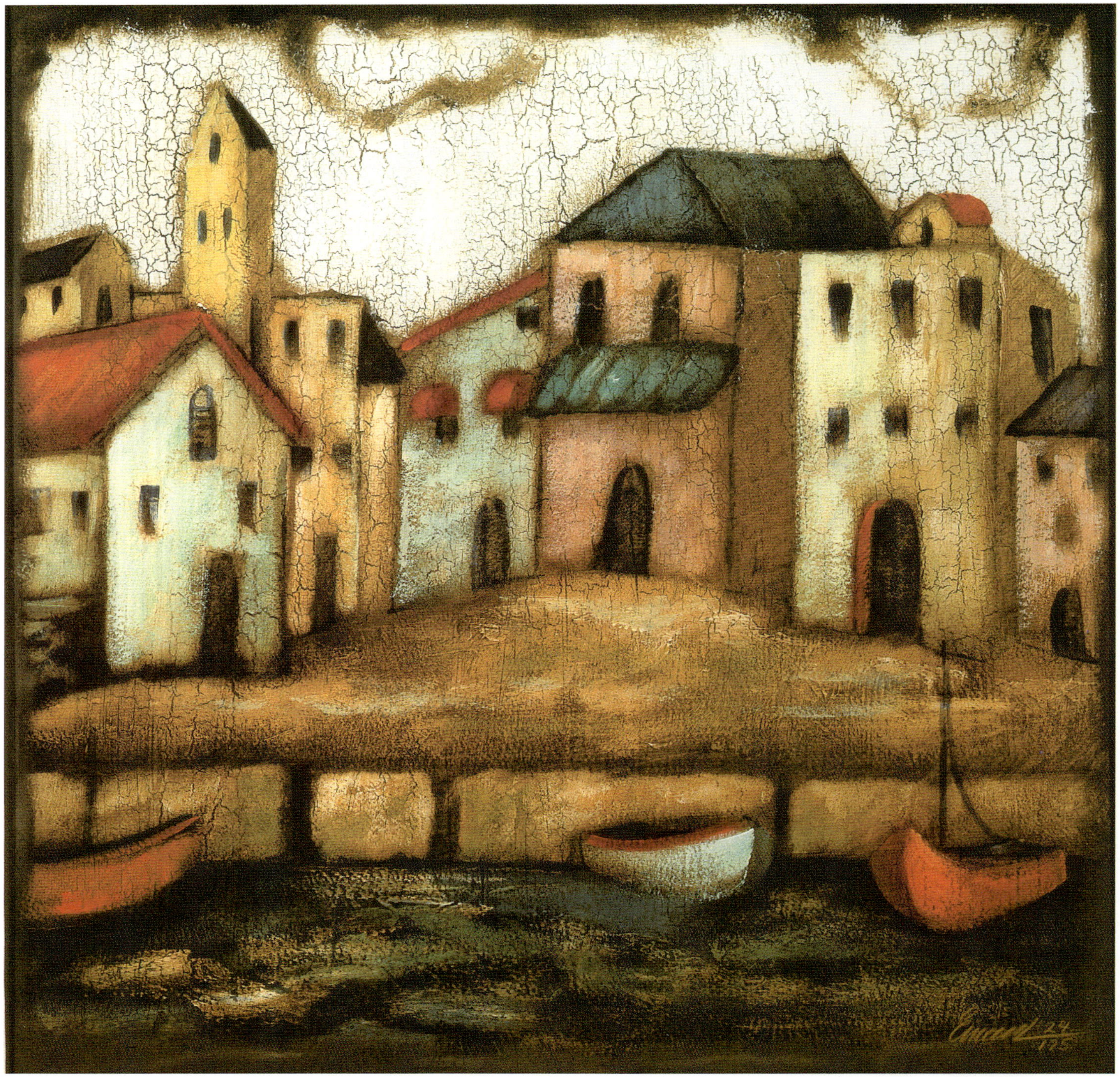

Casa X

Mixed Media on Paper 20"x20"

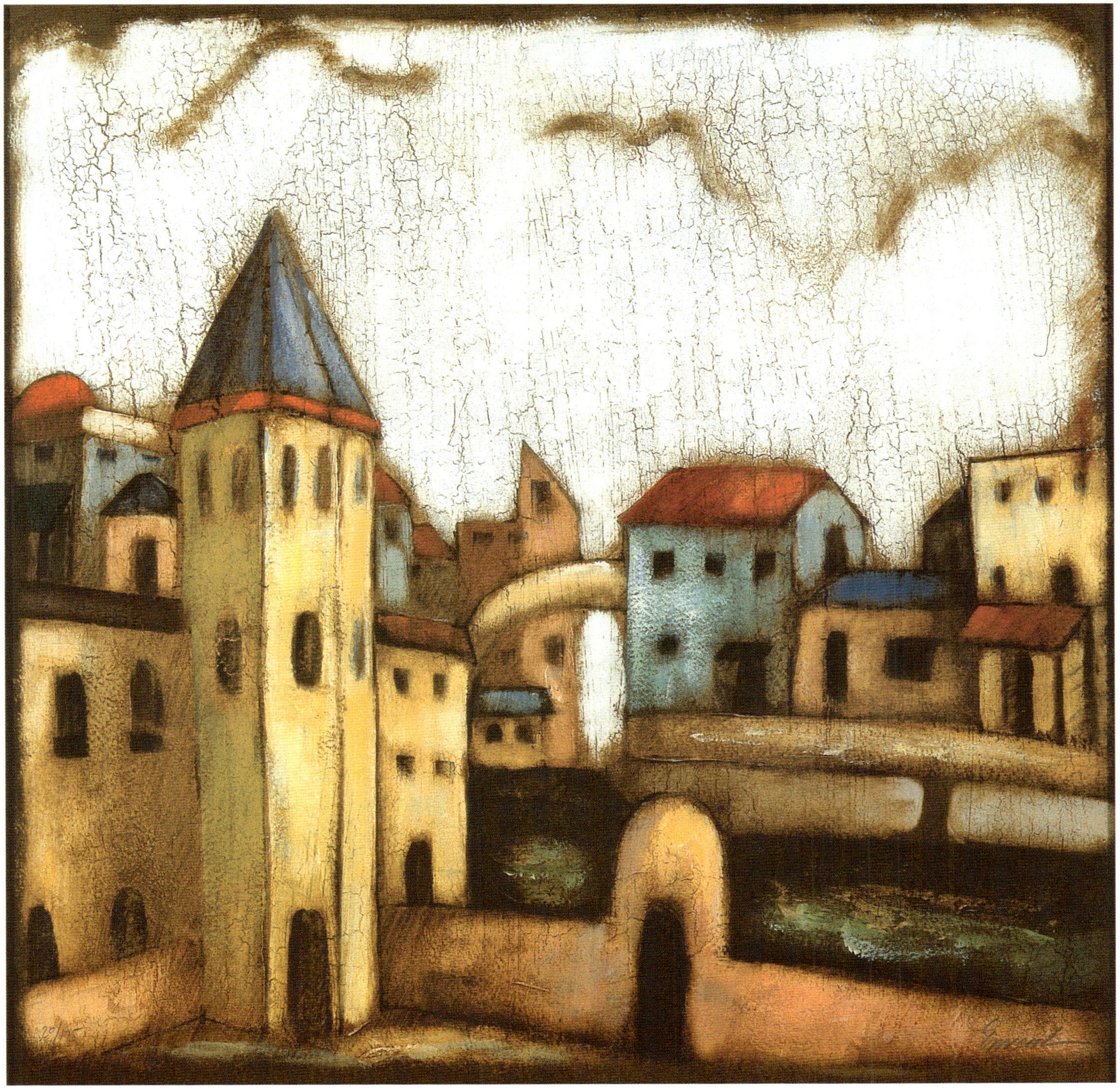

Casa XI

Mixed Media on Paper 20"x20"

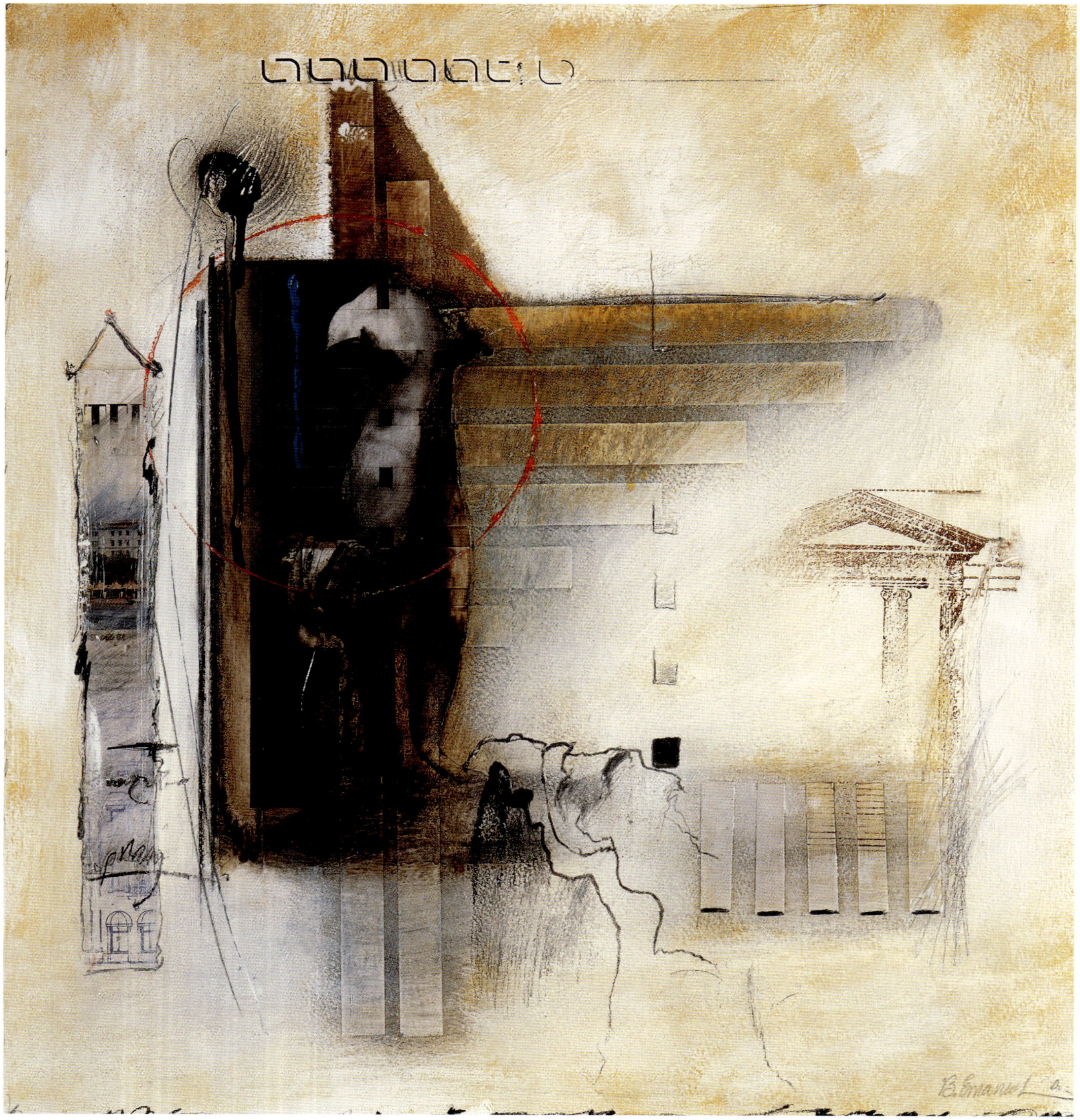

Appellation I

Mixed Media on Paper 18"x18"

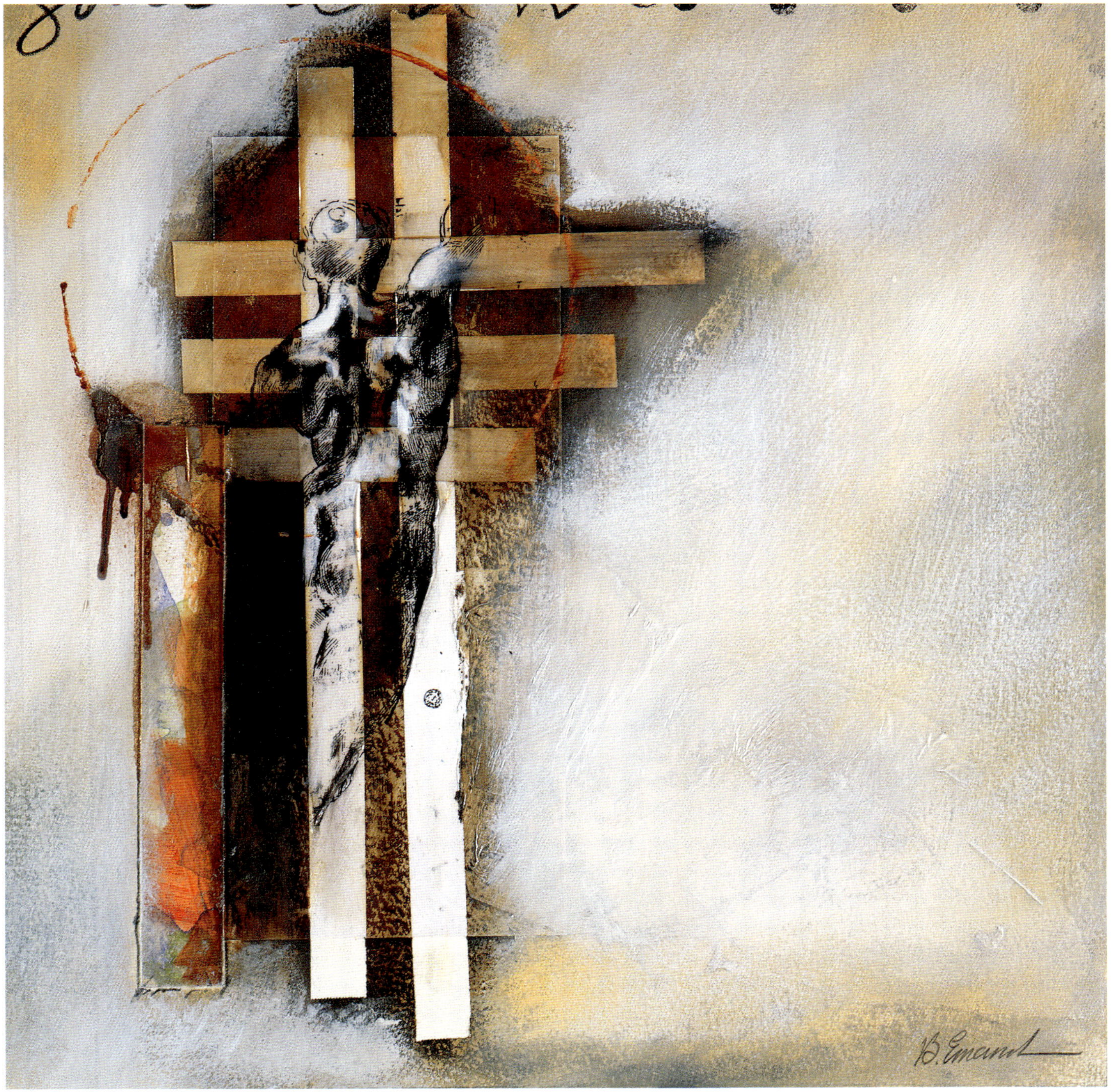

Appellation III

Mixed Media on Paper 18"x18"

The genius of Emanuel's paintings lies in his profound awareness of history and his ability to redefine the past in terms so original that they express **this time** and **this zeitgeist**. Like Conrad, he too is the pulse of this age. His art, while a glimmering reflection of the substructures of cultural and political realities that define the experiences of the twentieth century and its aesthetic outlooks, is also an aspiring aesthetic vision that establishes and seeks new vistas for the art of painting.

Above all, one deeply moving aspect of his cultural richness is how his art is always a substantiation of music. Musical harmonies are the roots from which his forms and colors spring. His paintings are woven by harmonic threads whose sensual flow transcends the forms of pure sensations. The melodic and the poetic potently merge in his abstractions, releasing deep-lying emotions that come from the inexplicability of being. "When I paint I am a song," says Emanuel "I am part of a rhythmic flow thrown into the river of time."

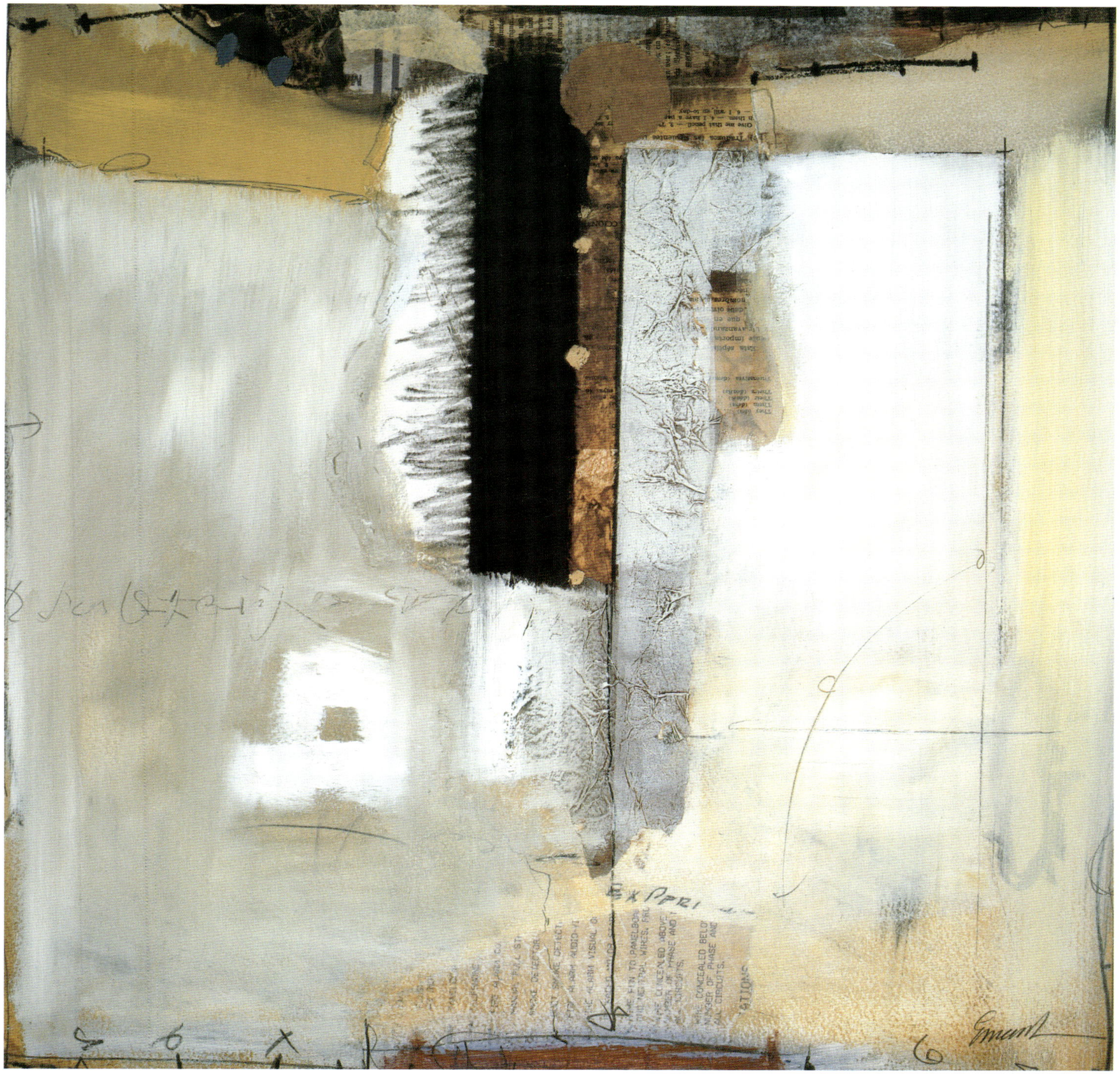

Ledger Line
Precis I

Mixed Media on Paper 20"x20"

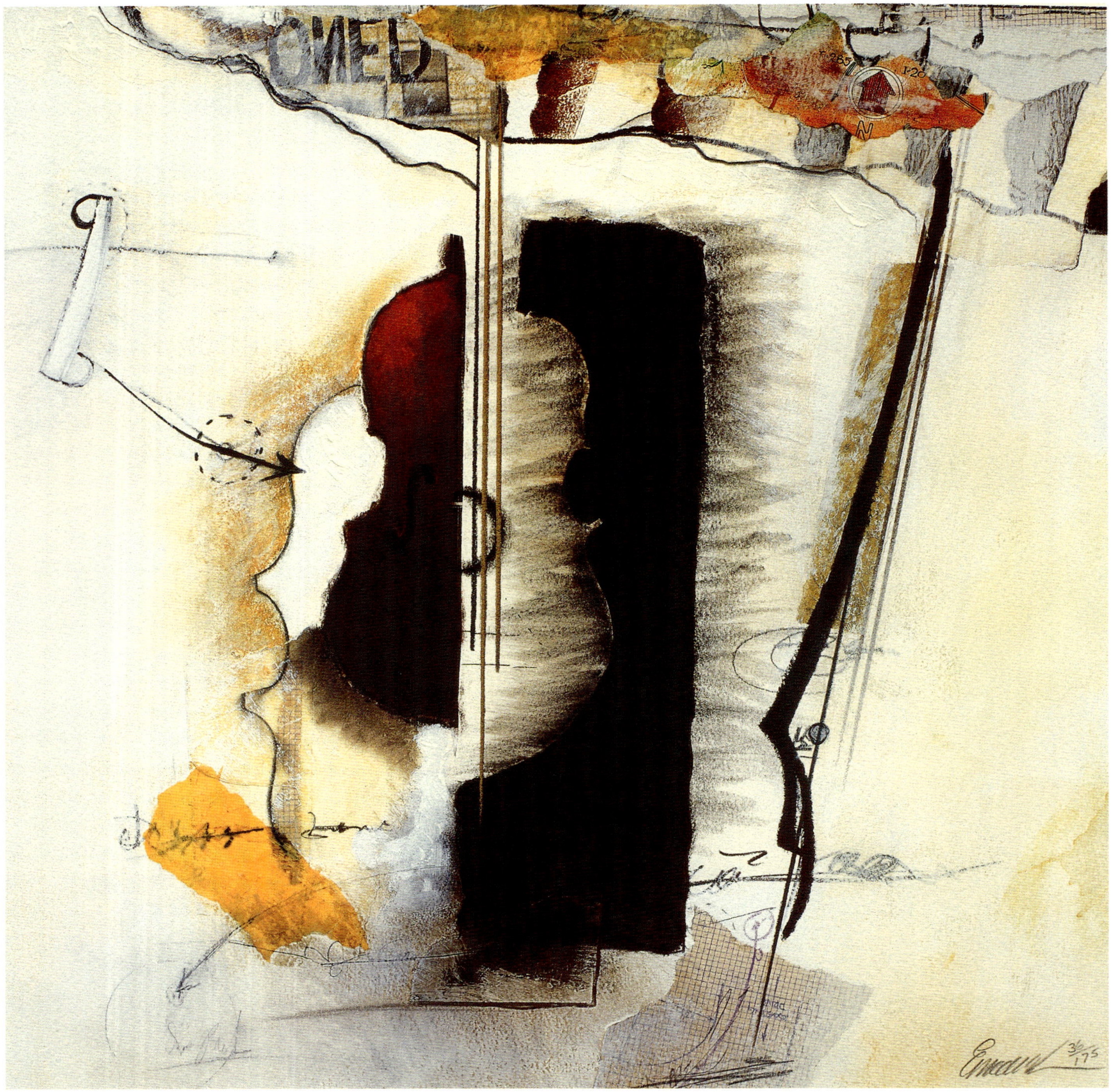

Ledger Line II

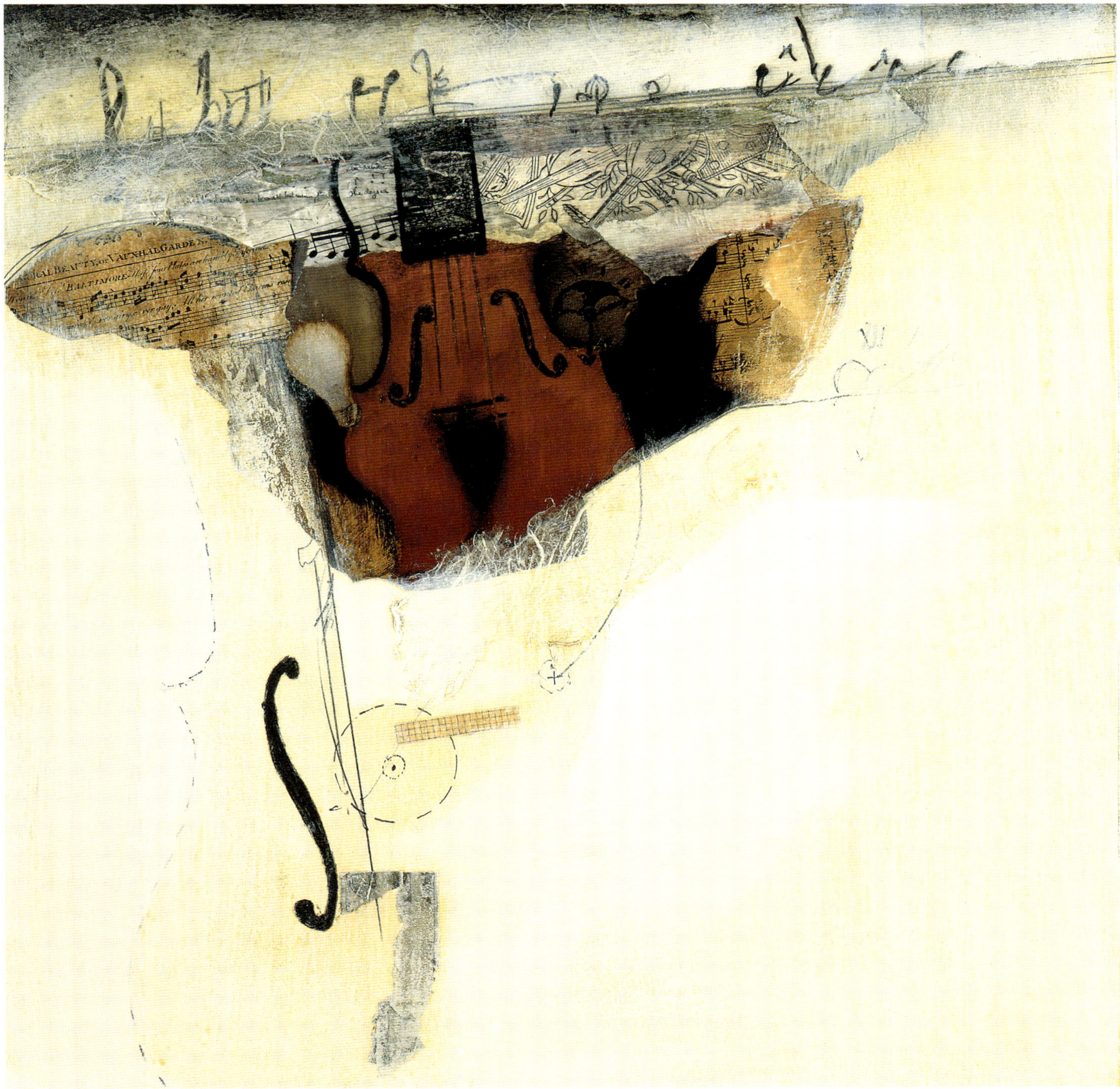

Ledger Line V

Mixed Media on Paper 20"x20"

Emanuel's art is a quest whose journey, as in the works of Robert Rauschenberg and Arshile Gorky, traverses the spectrum of modernist expressions and beliefs. Many of his works exemplify a passage from the bastions of modernist aesthetic into a sensuous imagination whose inwardness and immediacy is heartfelt. An example is his collage experiments where he embodies, on the one hand, the essence of contributions from masters such as Braque, Carra and Rauschenberg. On the other hand, he transcends their art by new visions of design and verbal content, establishing a new dialectic between language and art, past and present. Emanuel's collages are, however, more than a theoretical exercise or a decorative statement. They have a fervid emotional content that imparts a devotional quality found in icons of the Middle Ages.

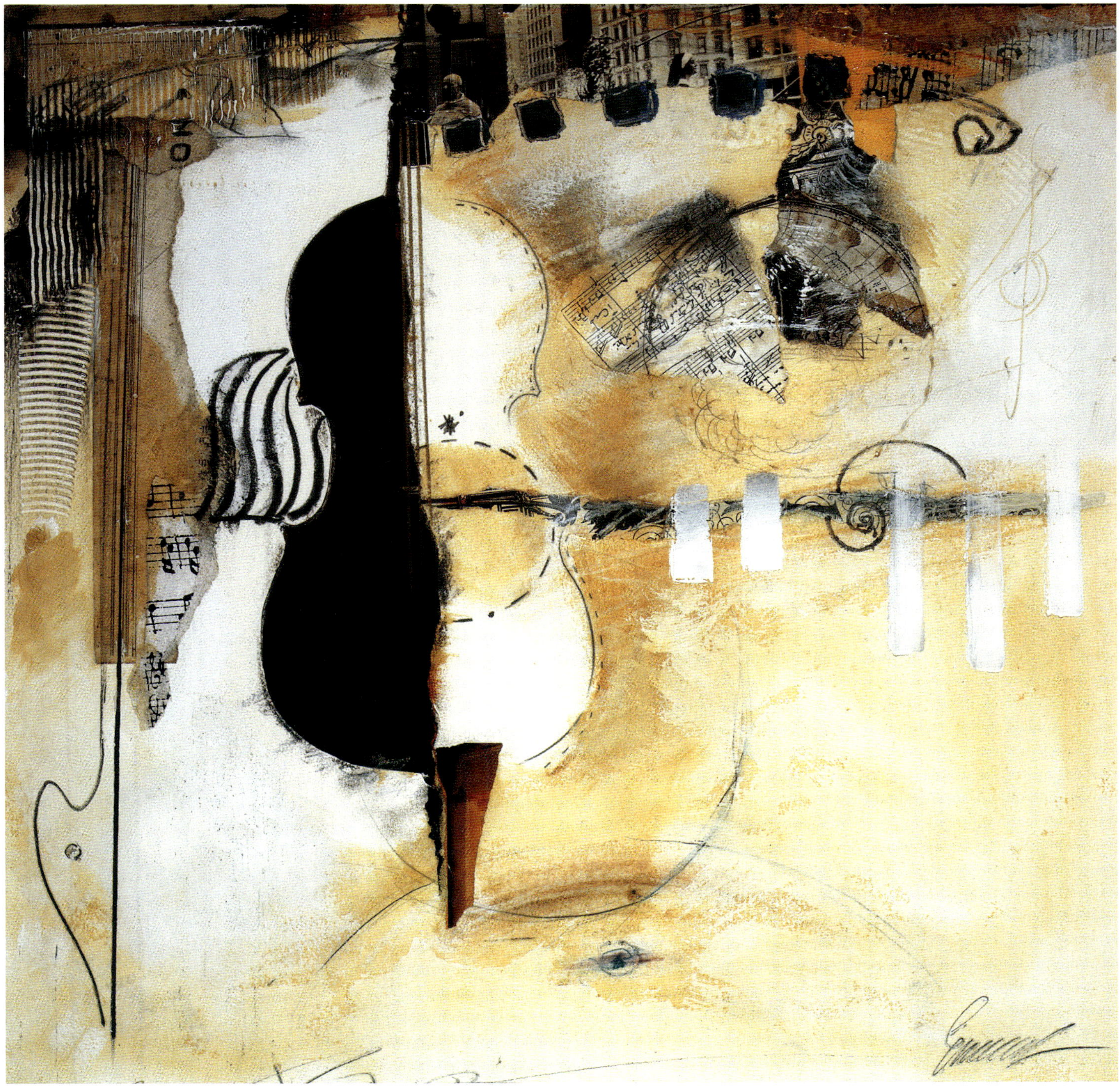

Ledger Line
Guitar Etude I

Mixed Media on Paper 18"x18"

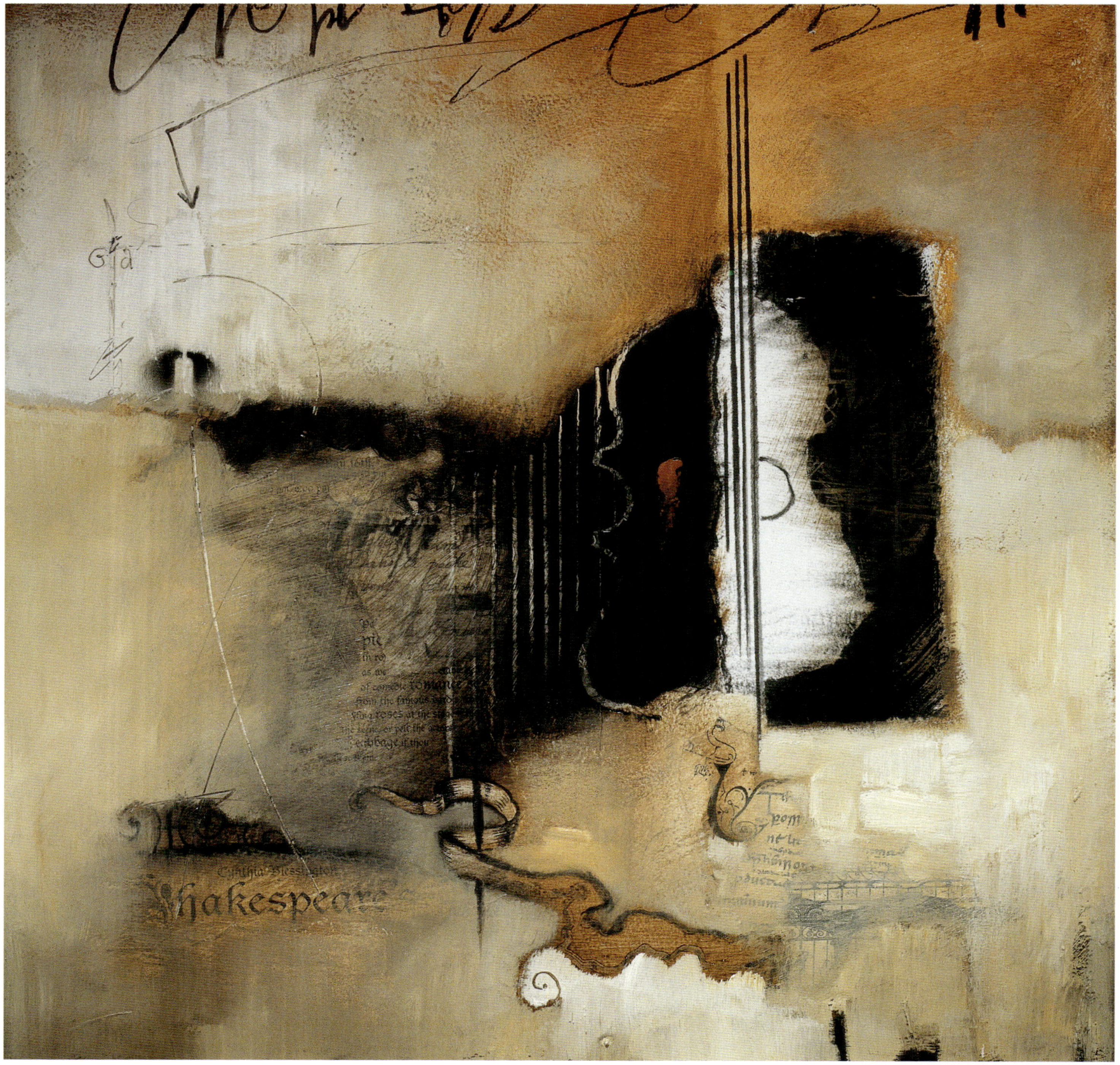

Ledger Line
Guitar Etude II

 Mixed Media on Paper 20"x20"

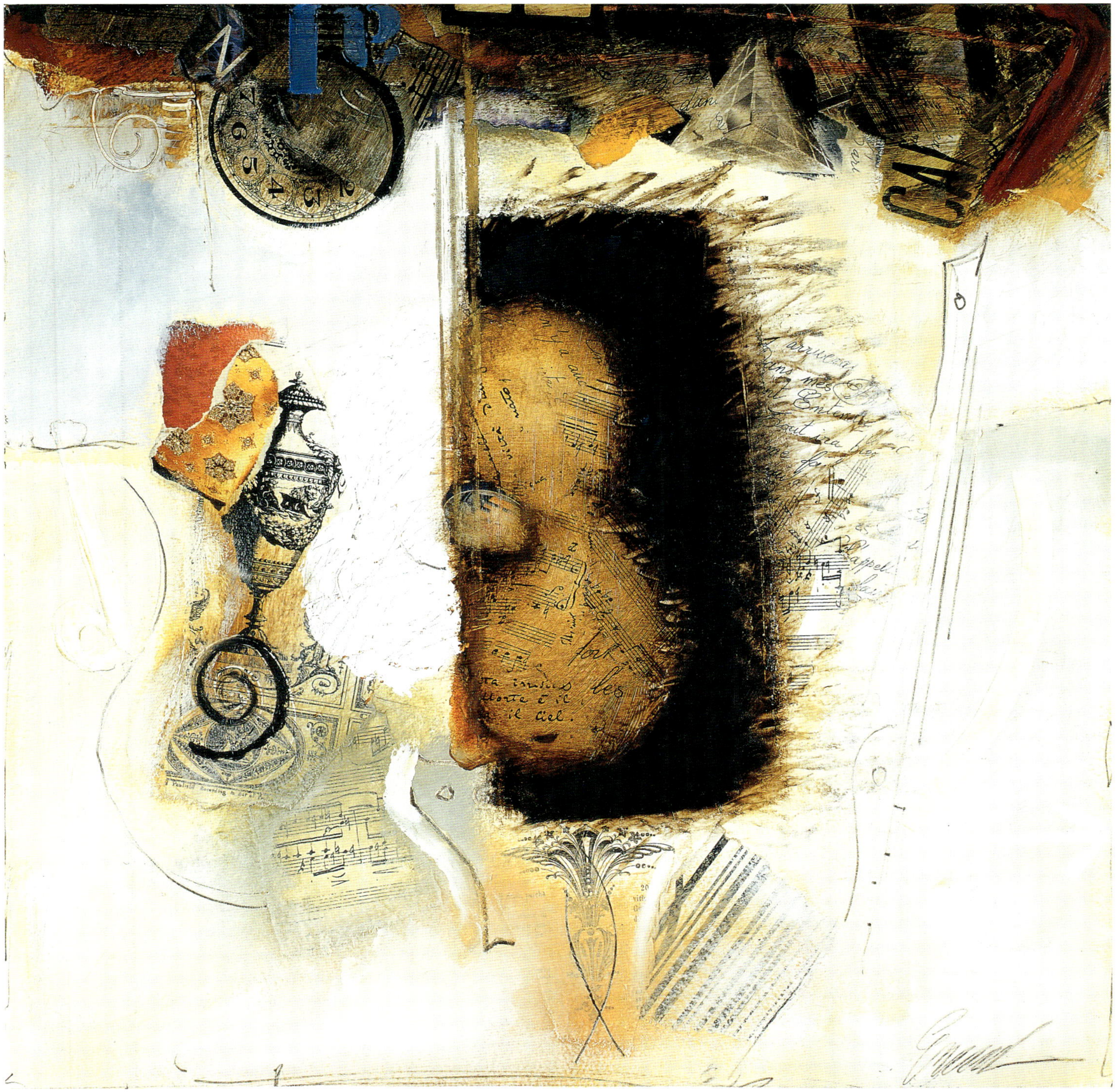

Ledger Line
Guitar Etude III

Mixed Media on Paper 20"x20"

Through skill, intuitive genius and an uncanny ability to interpret the domain of criticism and art history, Emanuel envisions spaces that emanate the powers of these manifold divisions. In this complex play of energies, his colors have a grandiloquent, operatic presence.

In work after work, and especially in the larger-scale abstractions, one striking feature in Emanuel's paintings is his use of color.

They rise with the dramatic immediacy of music and express diverse feelings that are often emphatic, sometimes romantic, even concrete and metaphysical. Anyone who has seen his abstractions recognizes that Emanuel's decisiveness of gestural acts, concomitant with his sense of coloring, overcomes the ambiguities of his abstract form and establishes a new and convincing logical framework of expression. In addition, the expanded size of his large-scale paintings affirms these principles irrevocably. Emanuel's abstractions, through the force of their coloring, breathe both the formation and the evanescence of materiality. In these paintings, platonic purity cohabits with tangible objects, making for scenes whose gravity is like Donne's poetry, always transferring and transmuting energies of the substantial world into new prophetic dreams.

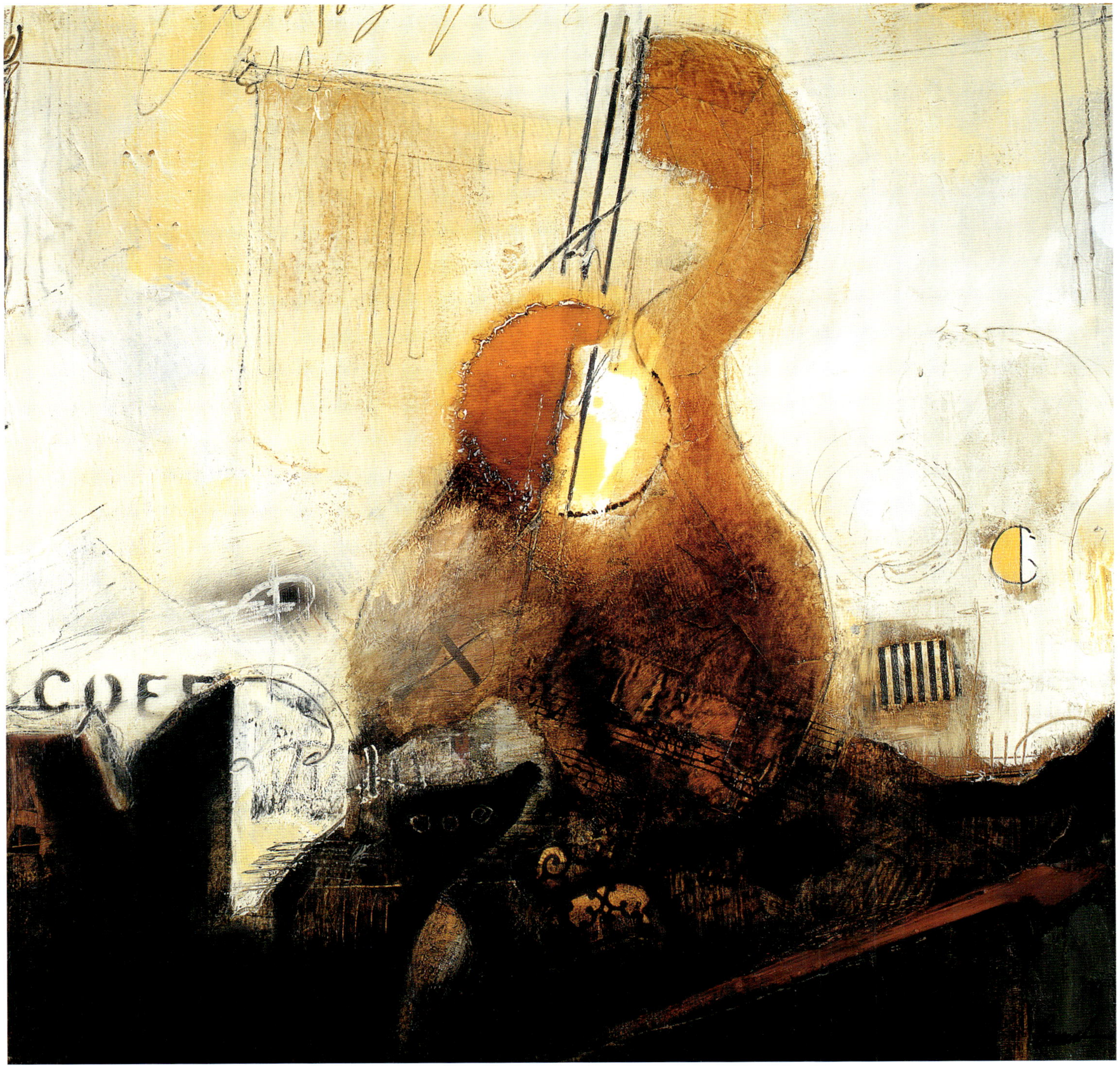

Ledger Line
Guitar Etude IV

Mixed Media on Paper 20"x20"

Like Rauschenberg's **"Combine Paintings,"** Emanuel's works often revolve around the question of representation in the modernist context. They are historical testimonies to the art of collage and yet unique because they are unburdened by borrowing. They may allude to a fabric of tradition, but they also easily point to and fixate on new psychological and philosophical perspectives. Emanuel's fondness to paint **en serie** creates a rational framework for the unfolding of infinite variations on any given theme. In series after series, a central idea is played out, radiating multiple visions of being and often undermining the central reality in favor of change and flux. This attribute, which is central to the postmodern expressions of late twentieth century art, is also manifested in his stylistic pluralism and diversity of expression which reveal his uncanny sensitivity to the multicultural context of the present age.

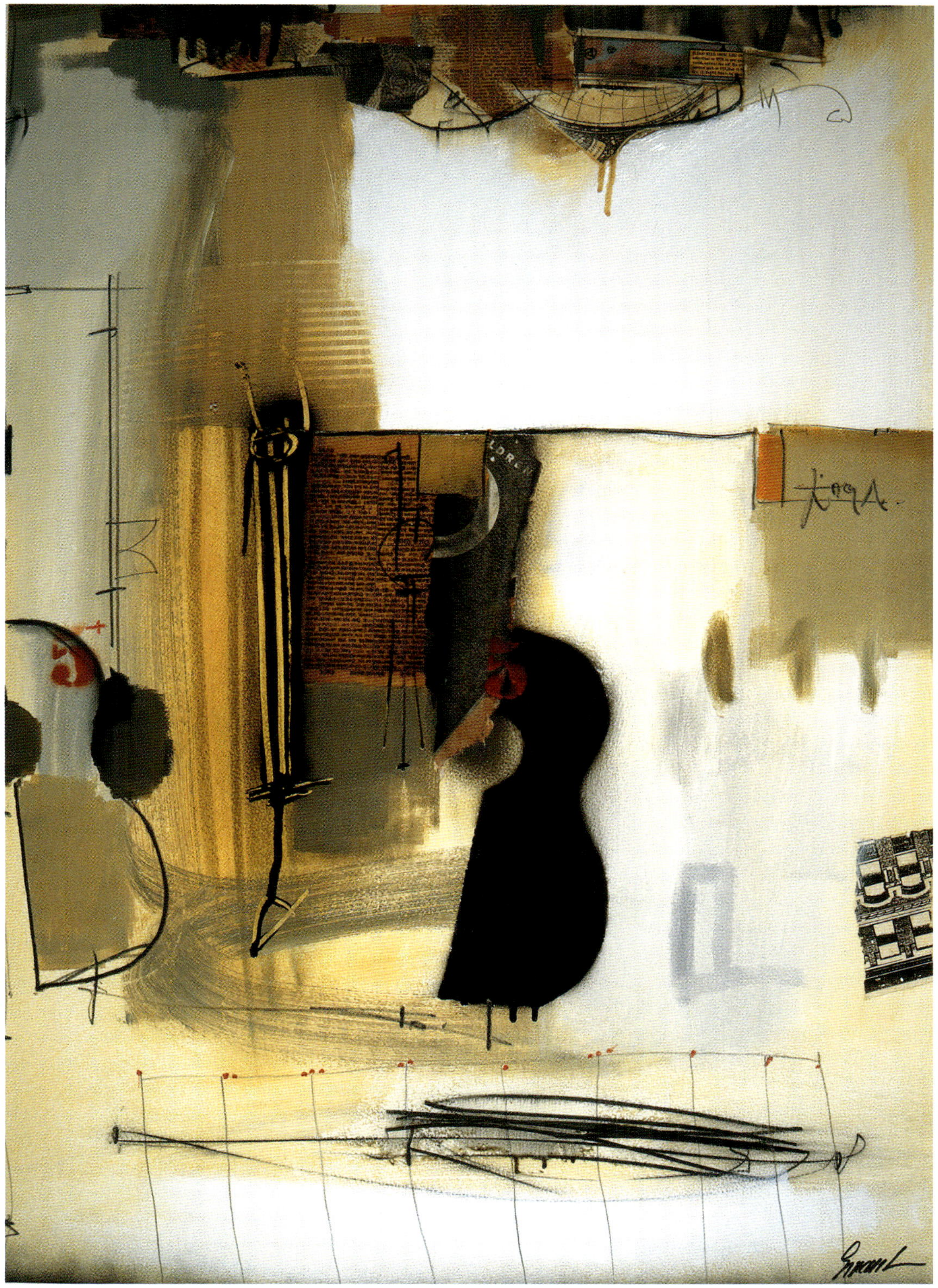

Ledger Line
Privia Eroica I

Mixed Media on Paper 24"x34"

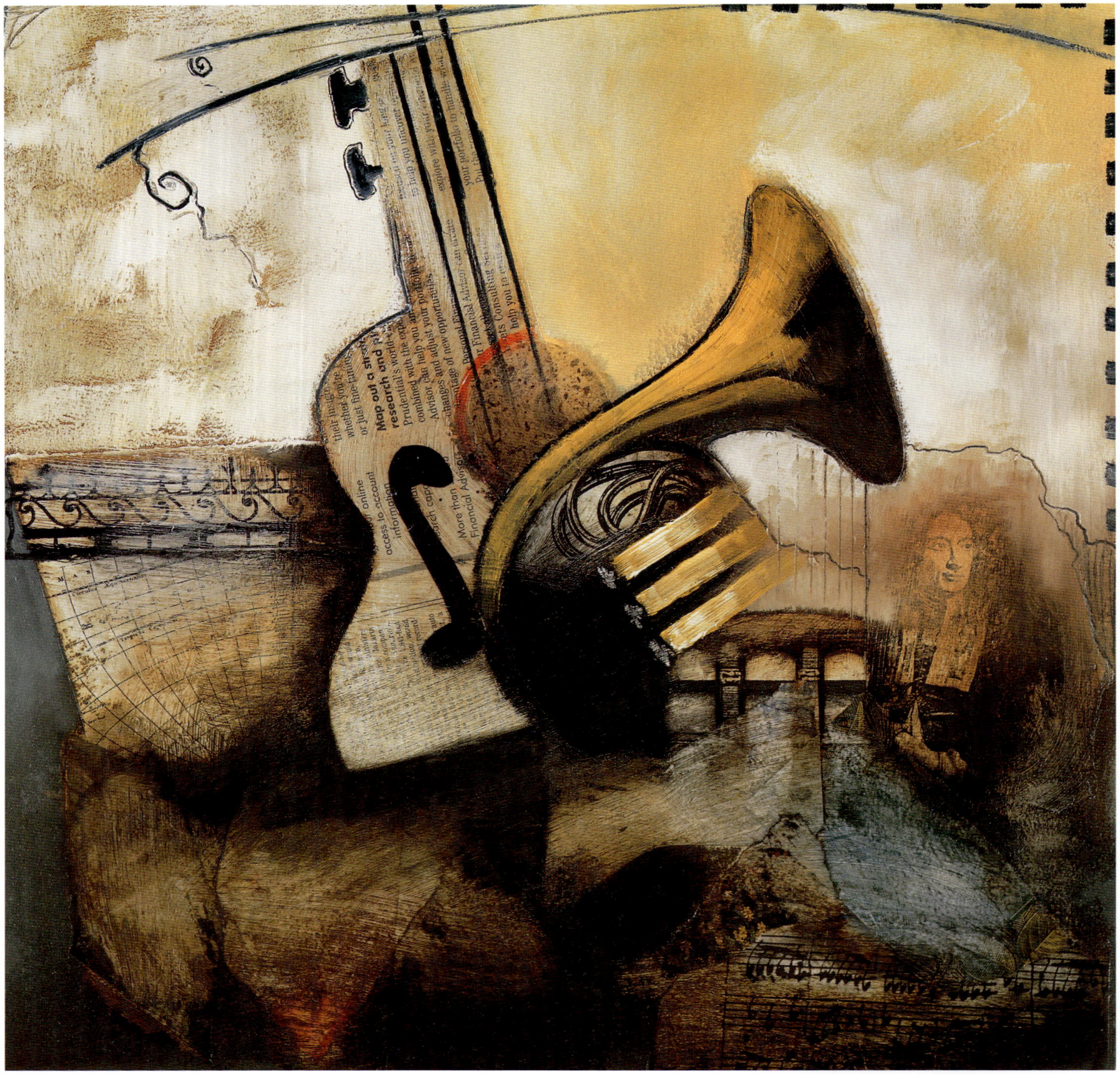

Concerto II

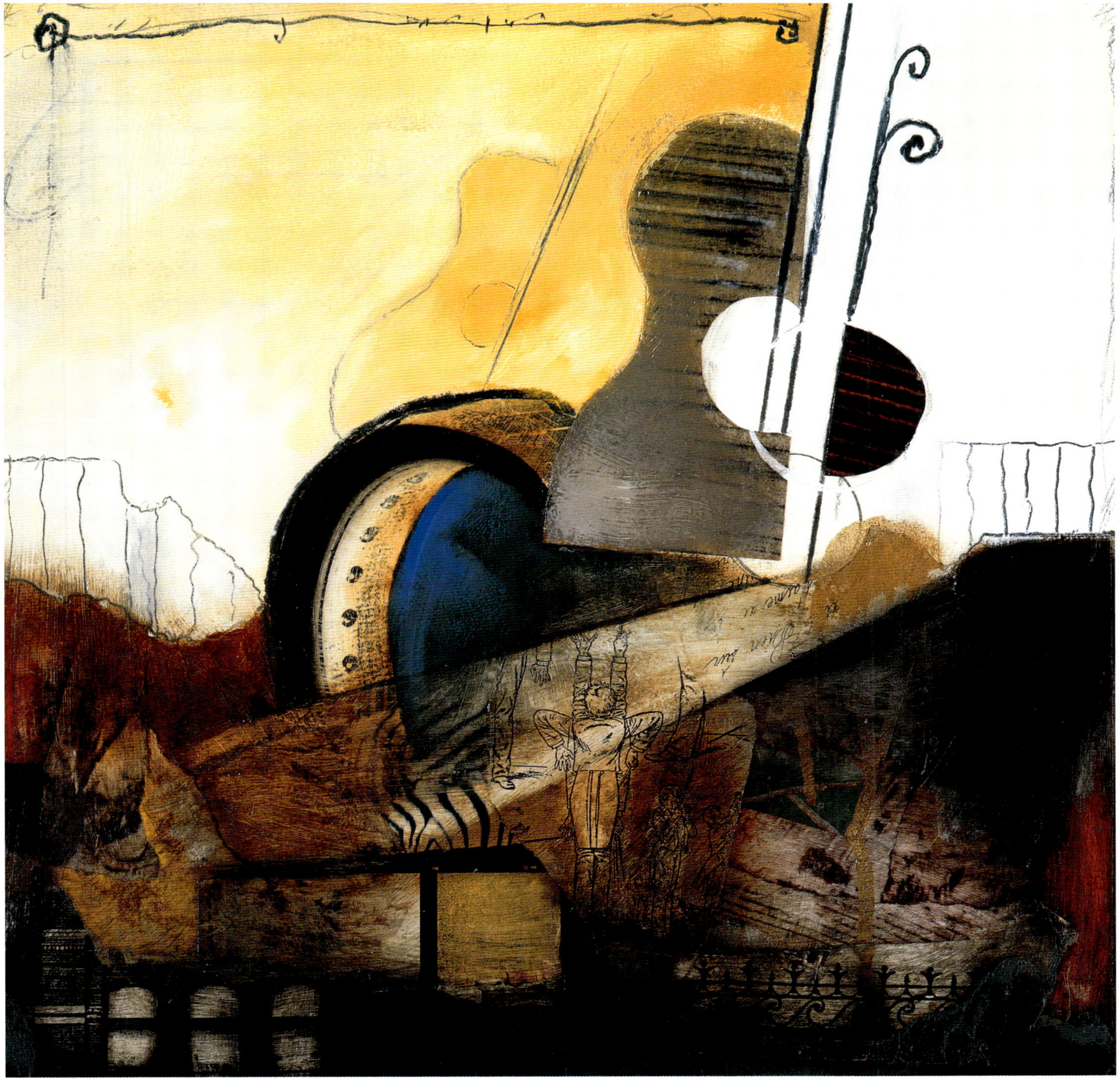

Concerto IX

Mixed Media on Paper 20"x20"

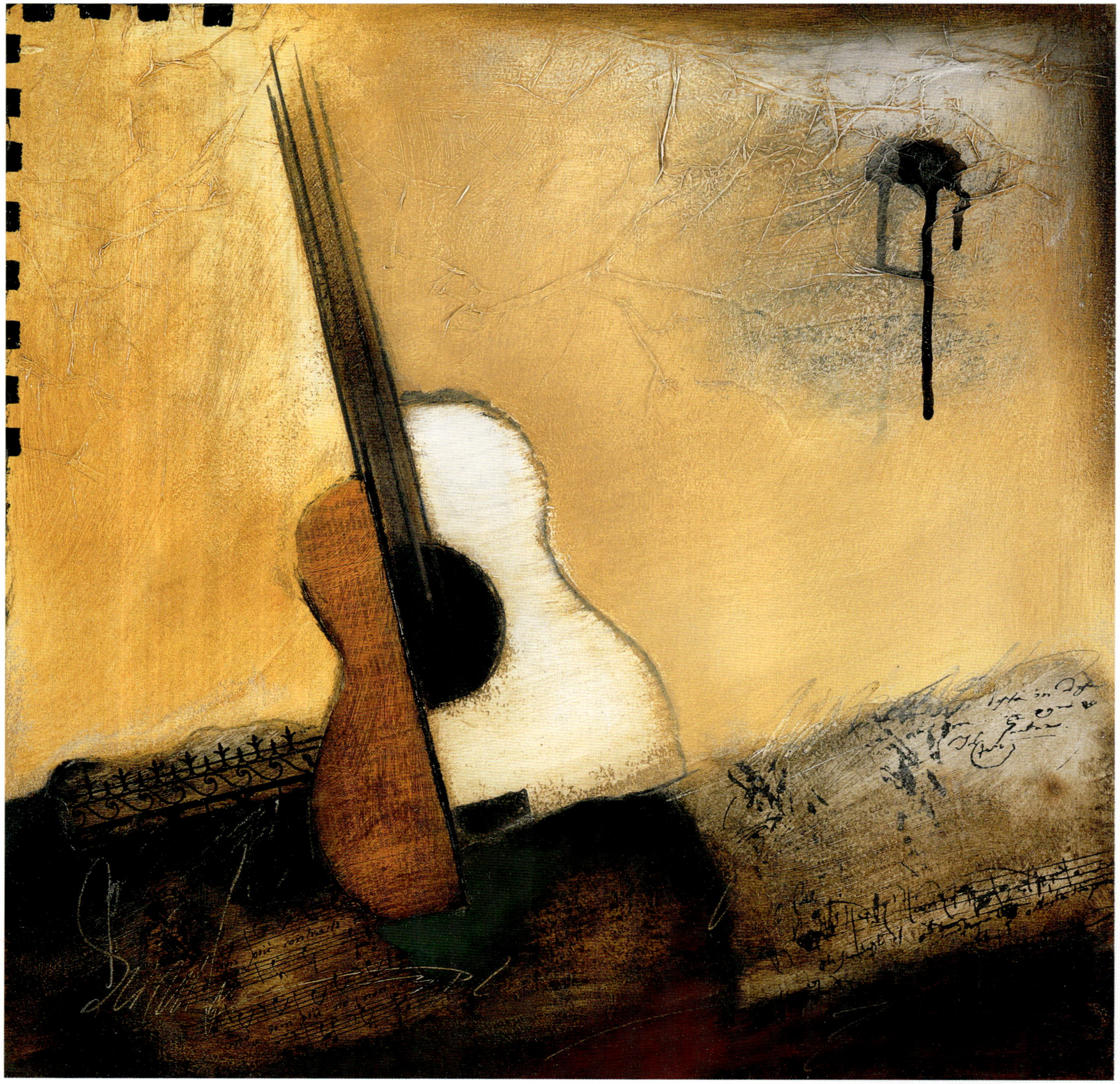

Concerto VI

Mixed Media on Paper 20"x20"

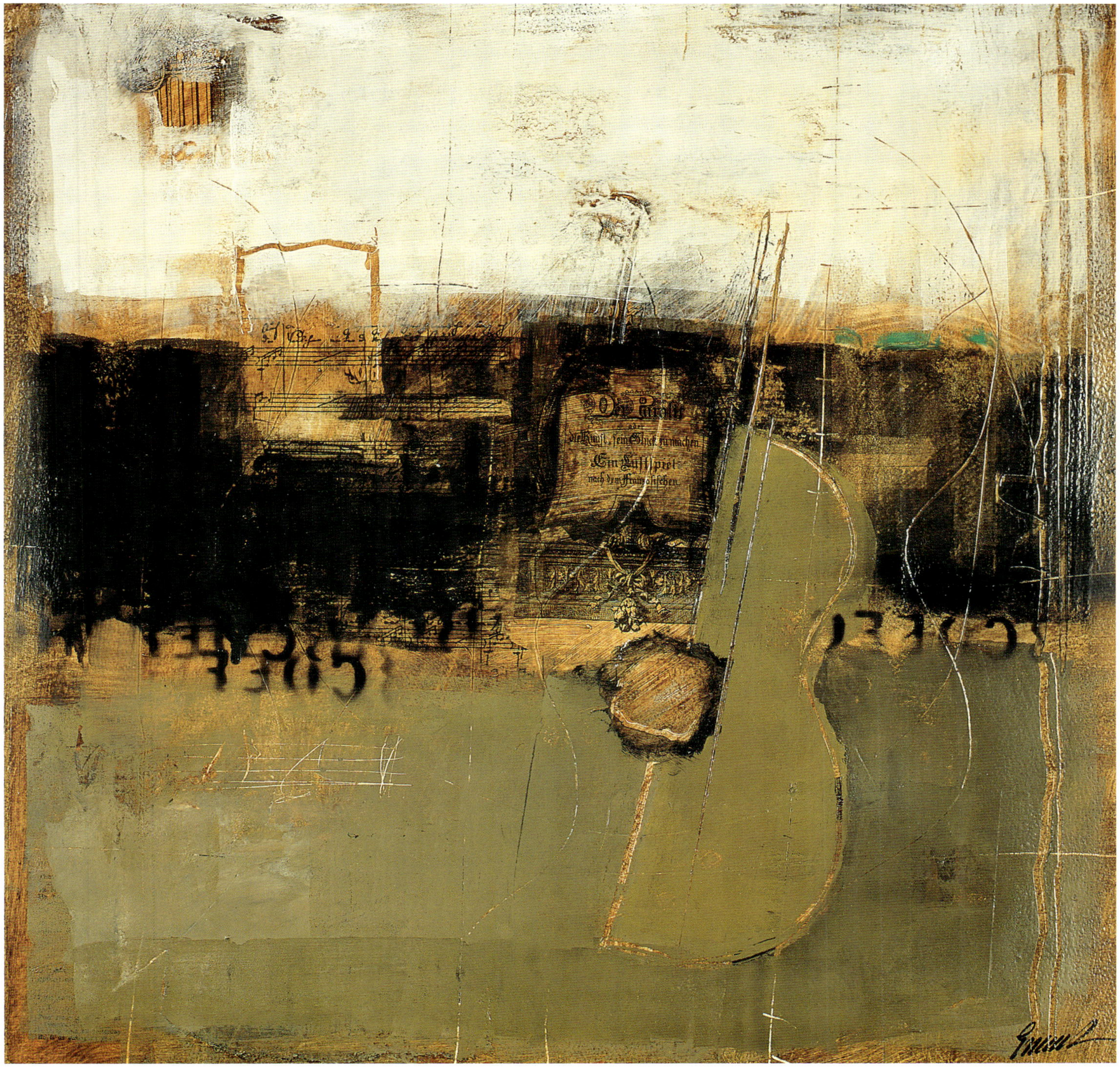

Concerto
Complicity Etude I

Mixed Media on Paper 20"x20"

Emanuel's sense of drama is unique. In the **"Hallycon"** series, the sense of drama and mystery that permeates the paintings derives from heightening the ambiguities of forms towards a lyrical and poetic tone. He composes masses with rhythmical movements, activating a momentum whose brooding lyricism is rich and luxurious. Like the theatre of Halcyon, this series is resolved to skepticism, passion and abandonment.

It turns the real into unbounded dreams and replaces meaning with complex sensory presence.

All of his works are touched by a full-blooded baroque magnificence, be they the darker, brooding sonnets of **"Hallycon"** or the complex witticisms of **"Orchestration."** In **"Orchestration,"** the spaces are perforated with discordant assemblies whose tonalities and unstable relationships heighten the dramatic impact of the paintings.

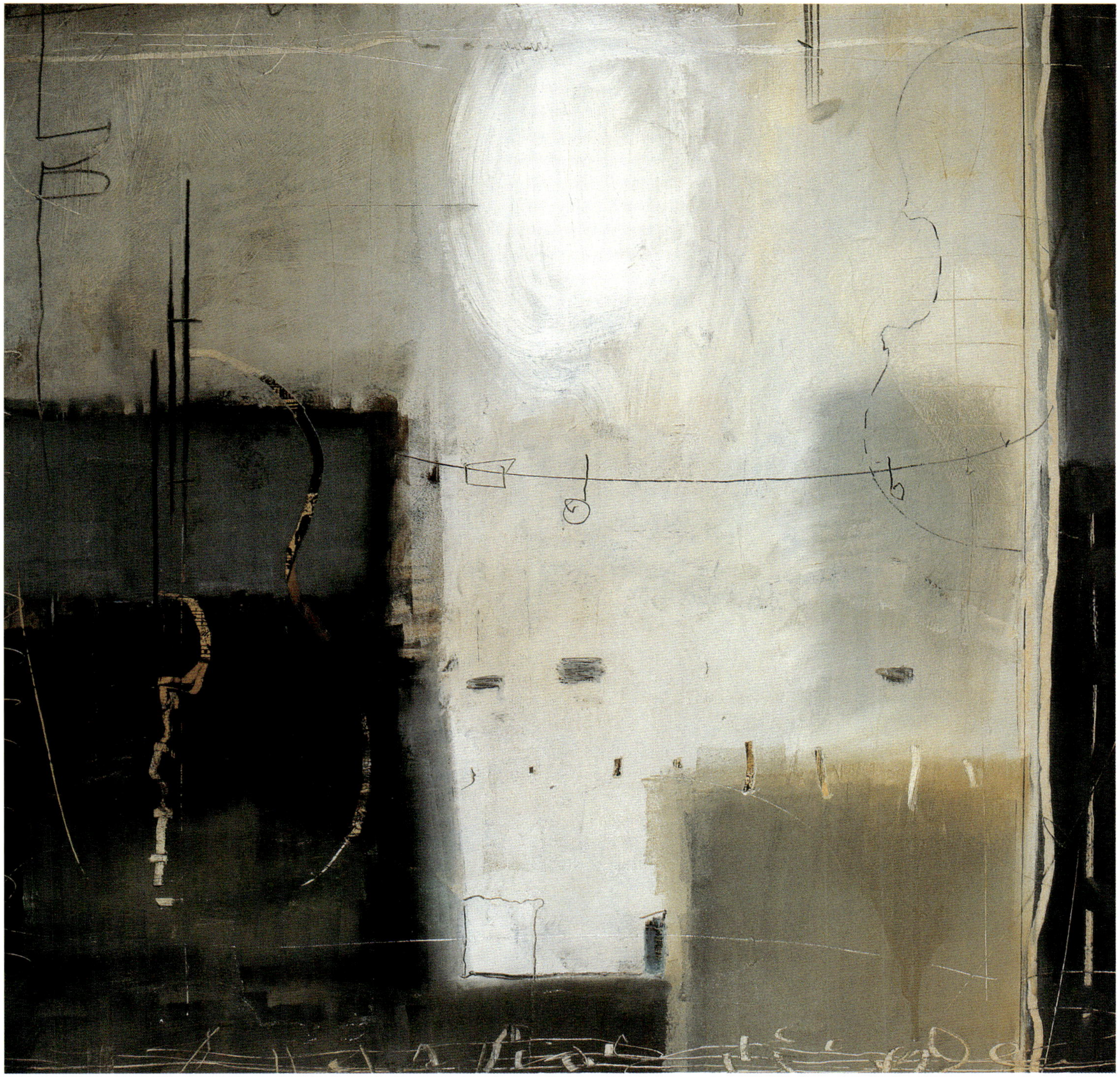

Concerto
Complicity Etude II

Mixed Media on Paper 20"x20"

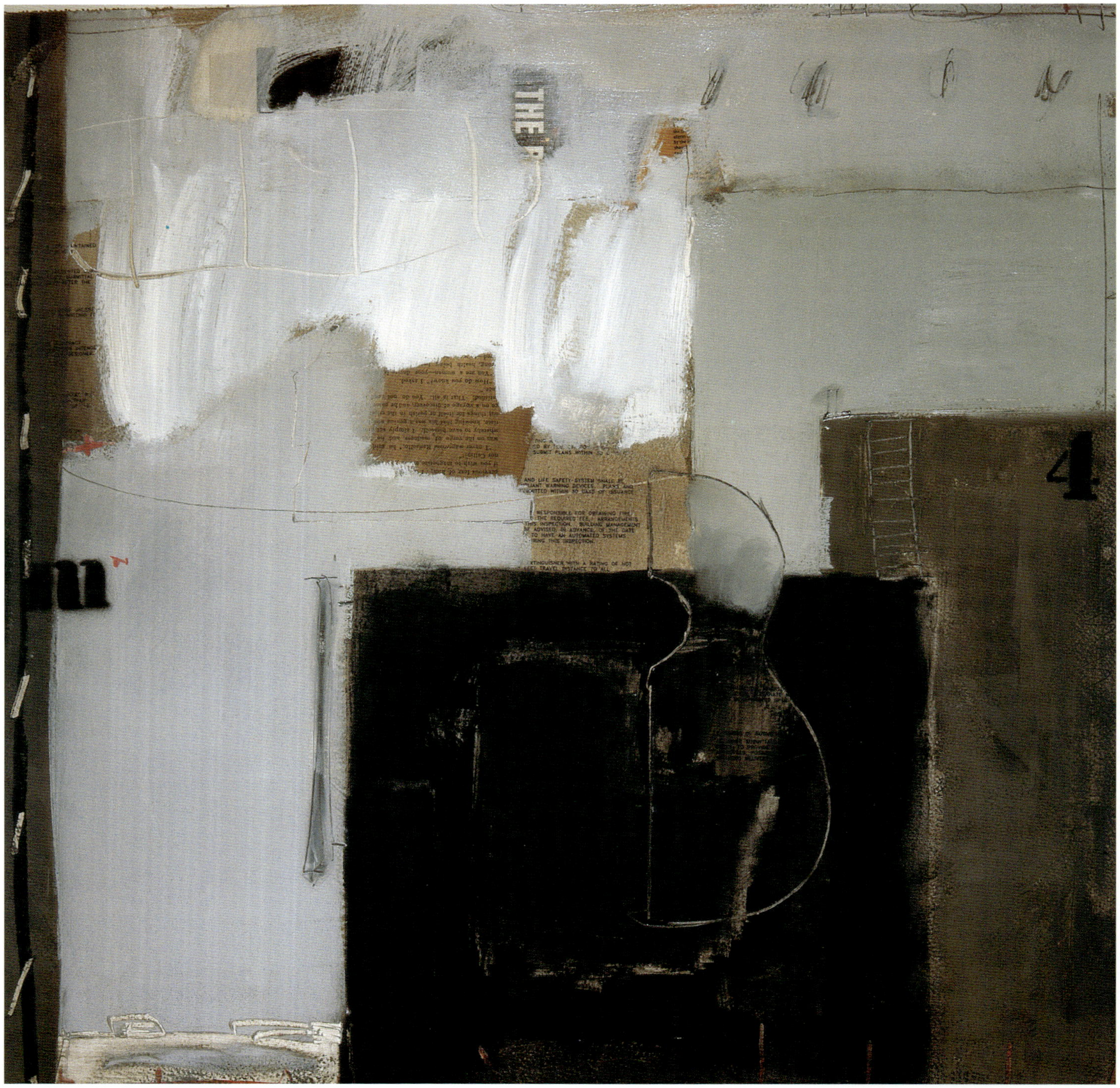

Concerto
Complicity Etude III

Mixed Media on Paper 20"x20"

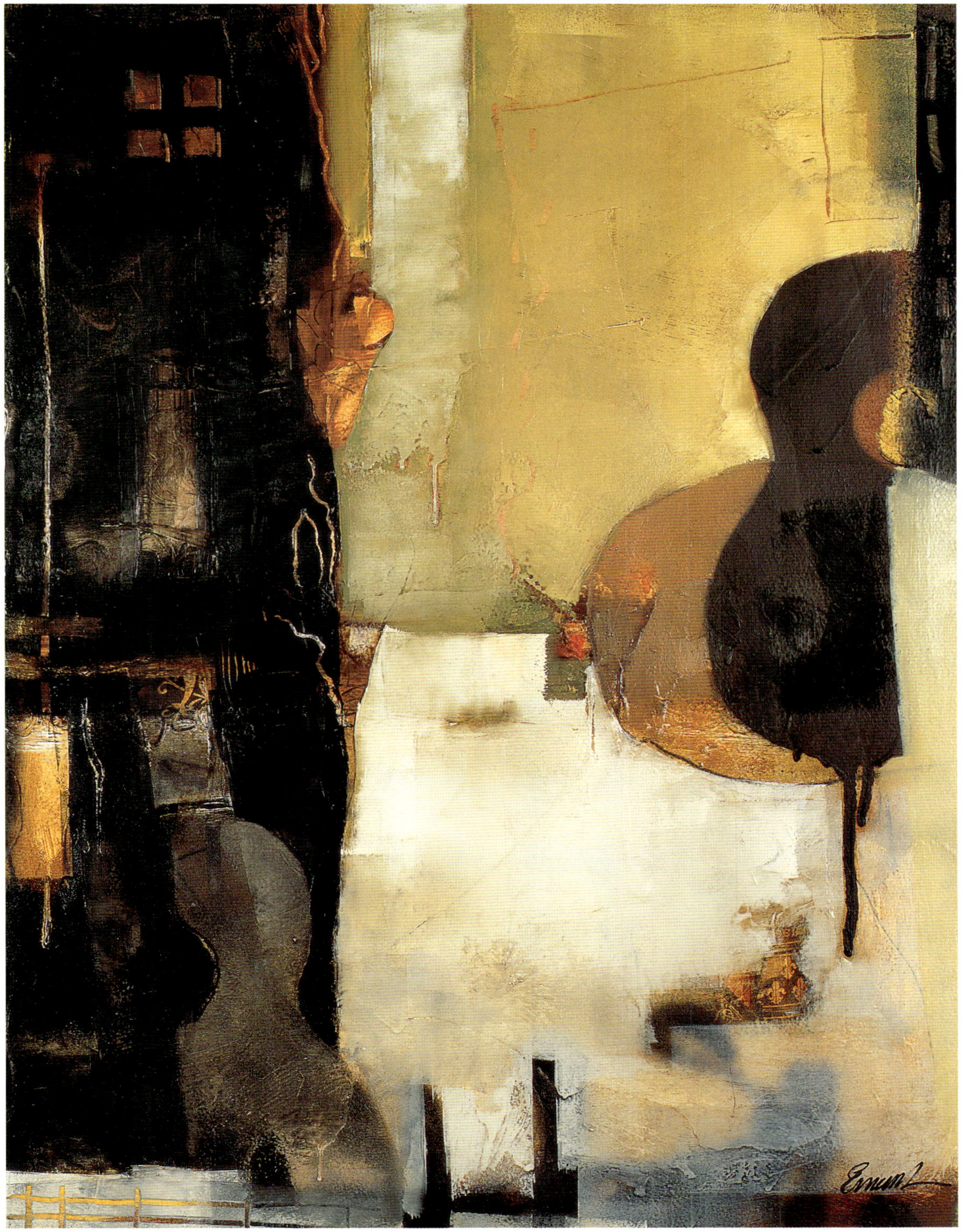

Concerto
Complicity Etude IV

Mixed Media on Paper 18"x24"

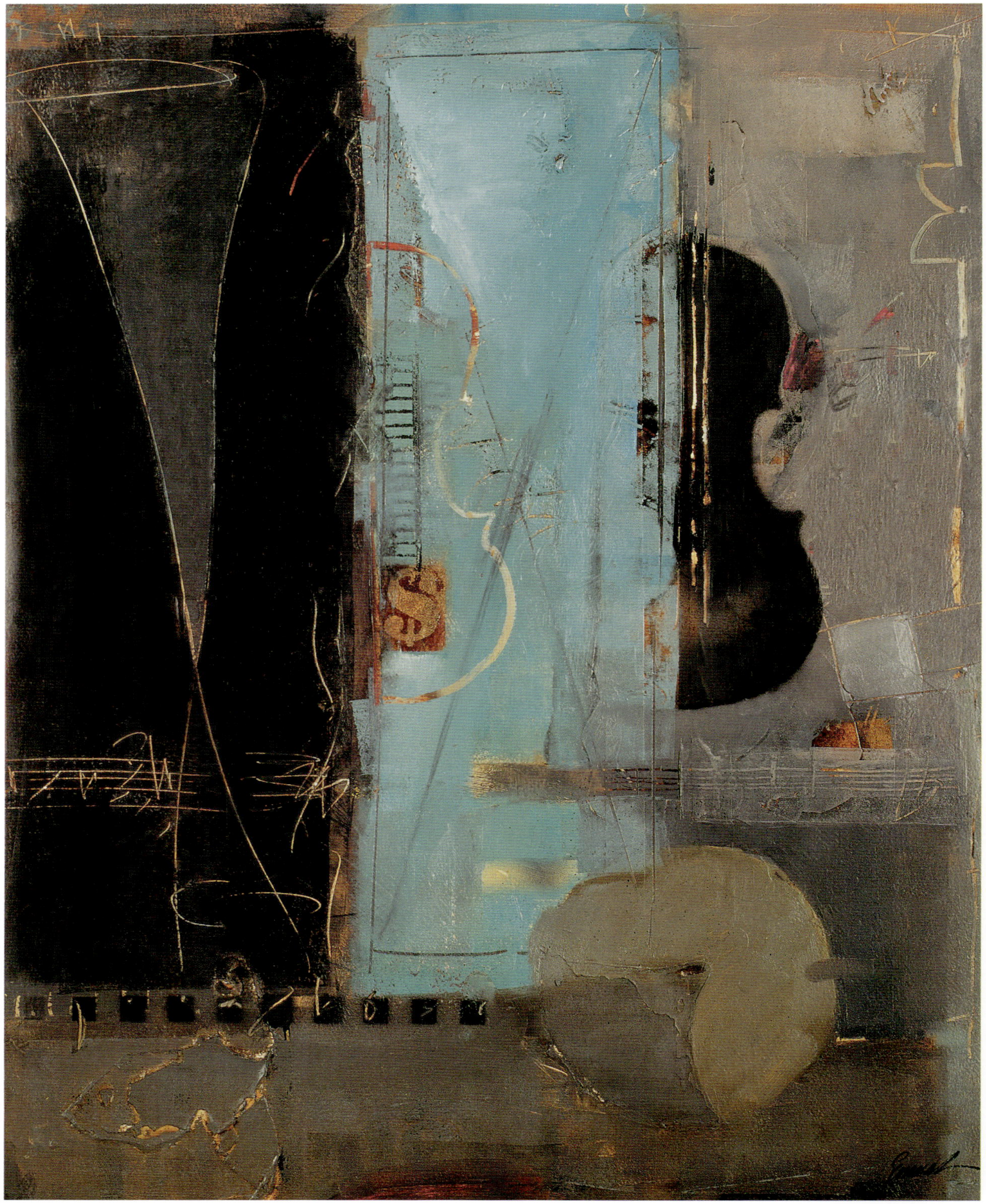

Concerto
Complicity Etude V

Mixed Media on Paper 18"x24"

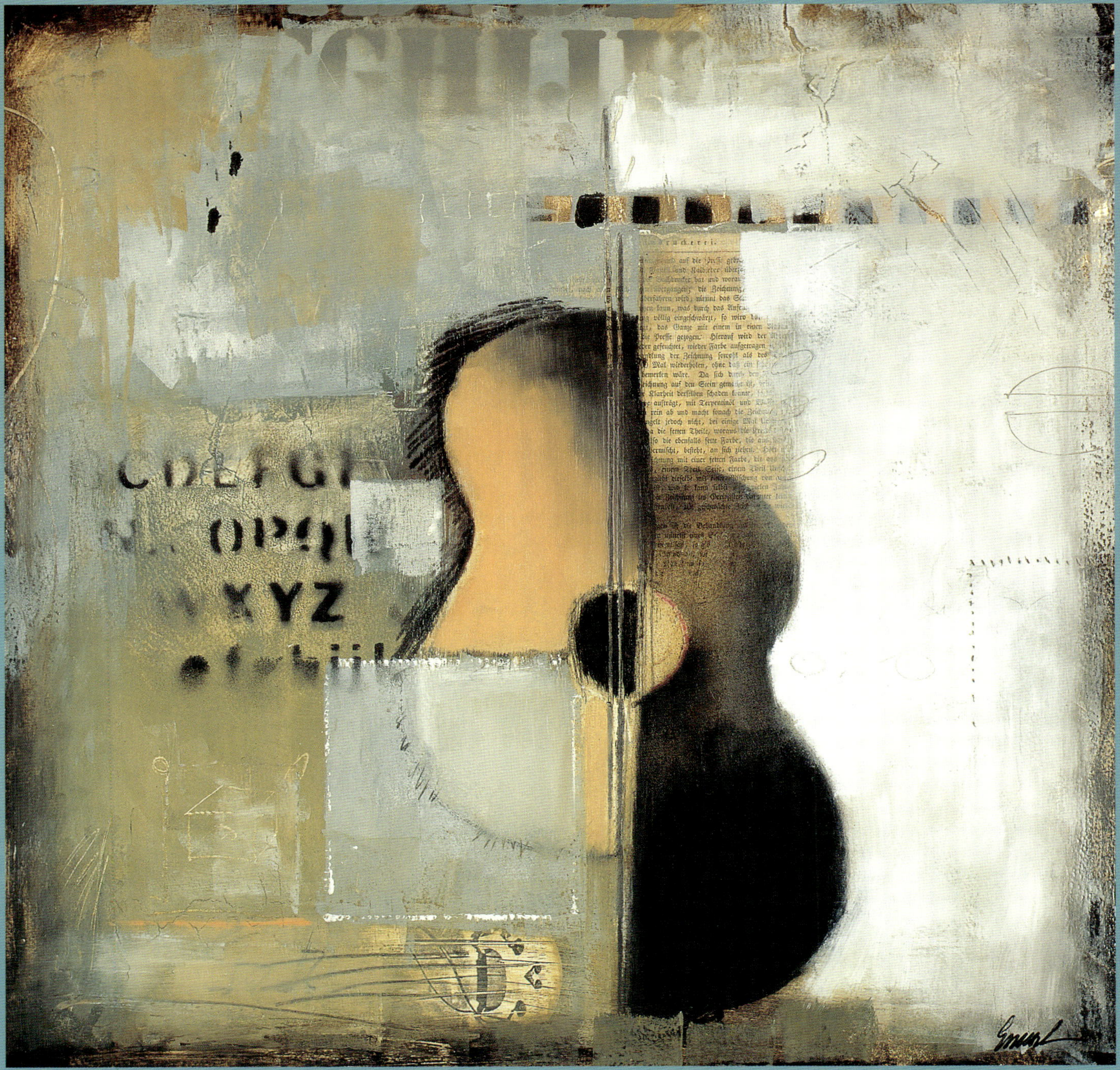

Concerto
Complicity Etude VI

Mixed Media on Paper 24"x24"

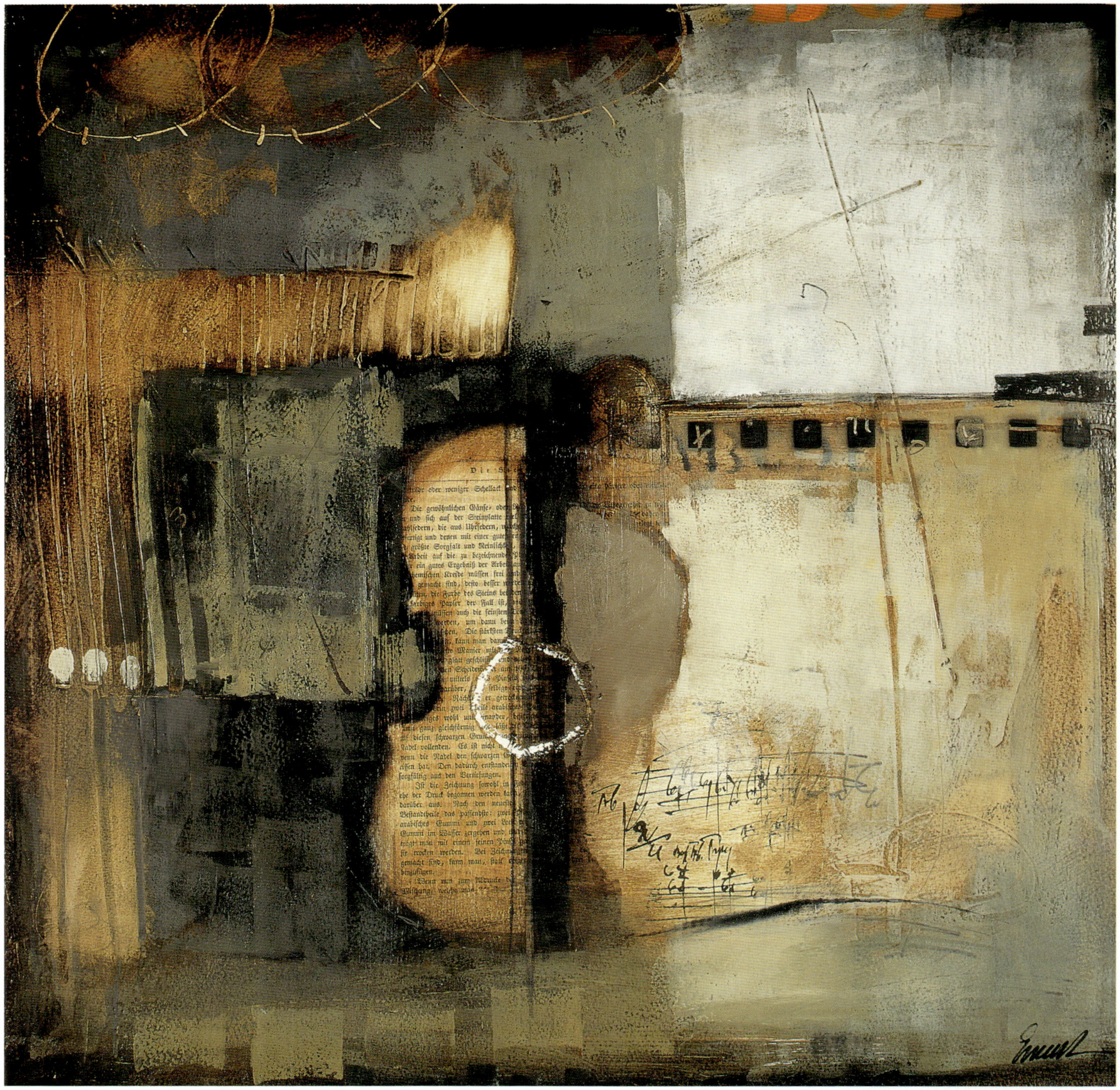

Concerto
Complicity Etude VII

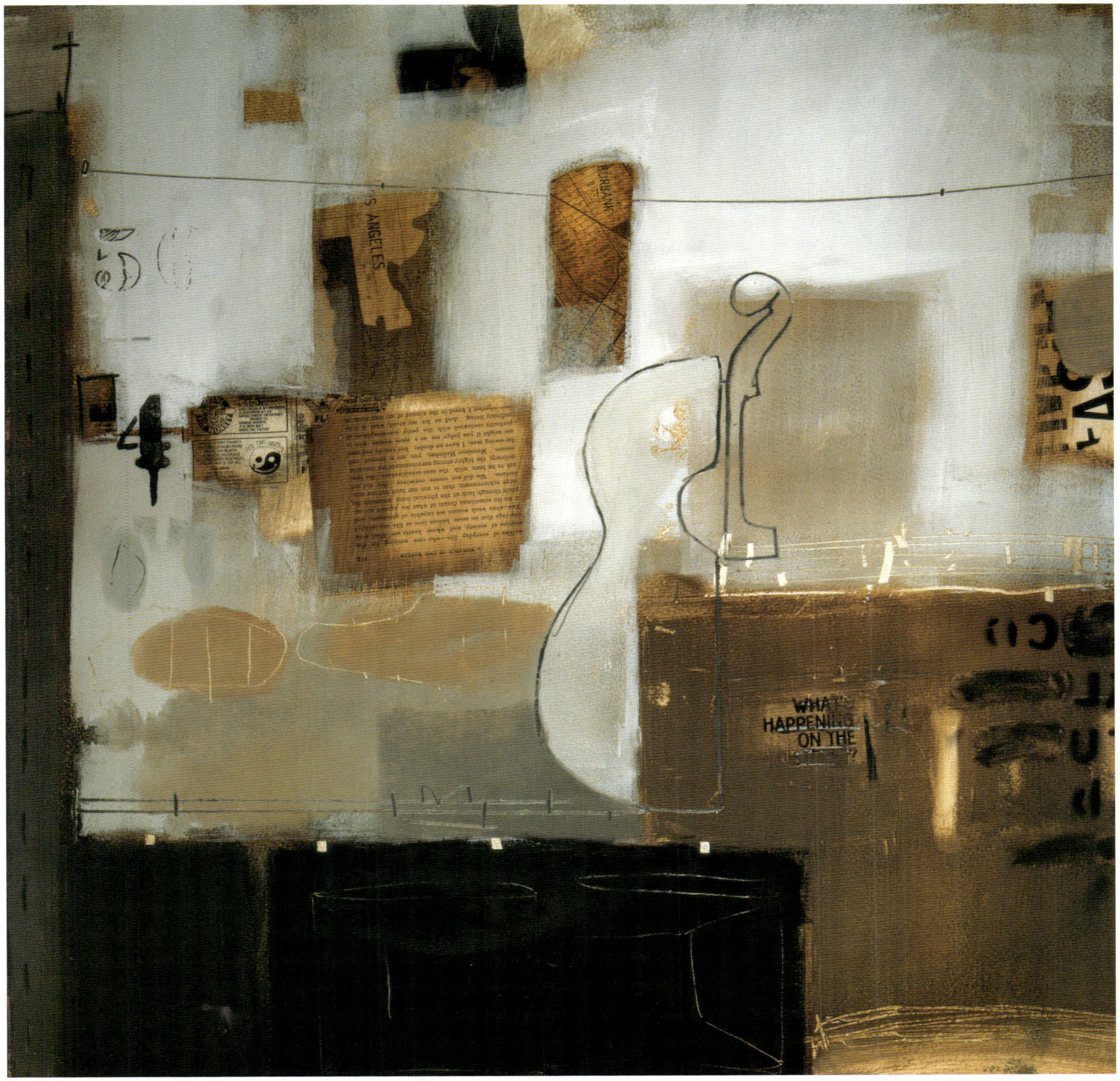

Concerto
Complicity Etude VIII

Mixed Media on Paper 20"x20"

The term that best defines Emanuel's modernist sensibilities is pictorial maturity. All of his compositions have a final iridescence of vision. Each element is so firmly grounded that the viewer cannot imagine revisions. The academic and the new blend so seamlessly that the final work is always a presentation of Emanuel's genius rather than a re-presentation of earlier ideas and forms. Even when he is dealing with earlier modernist styles, as in the collage or futurist formulations, he generates a new style—always resolving the uncertainties of the earlier forms and robustly sorting out the relevant from the irrelevant regarding his own life and age. His art brings conviction and is ardent in its aesthetic proclamations. In every painting, the forms are suited and adapted to a grander compositional scheme, working in concord toward a unified and resolute message.

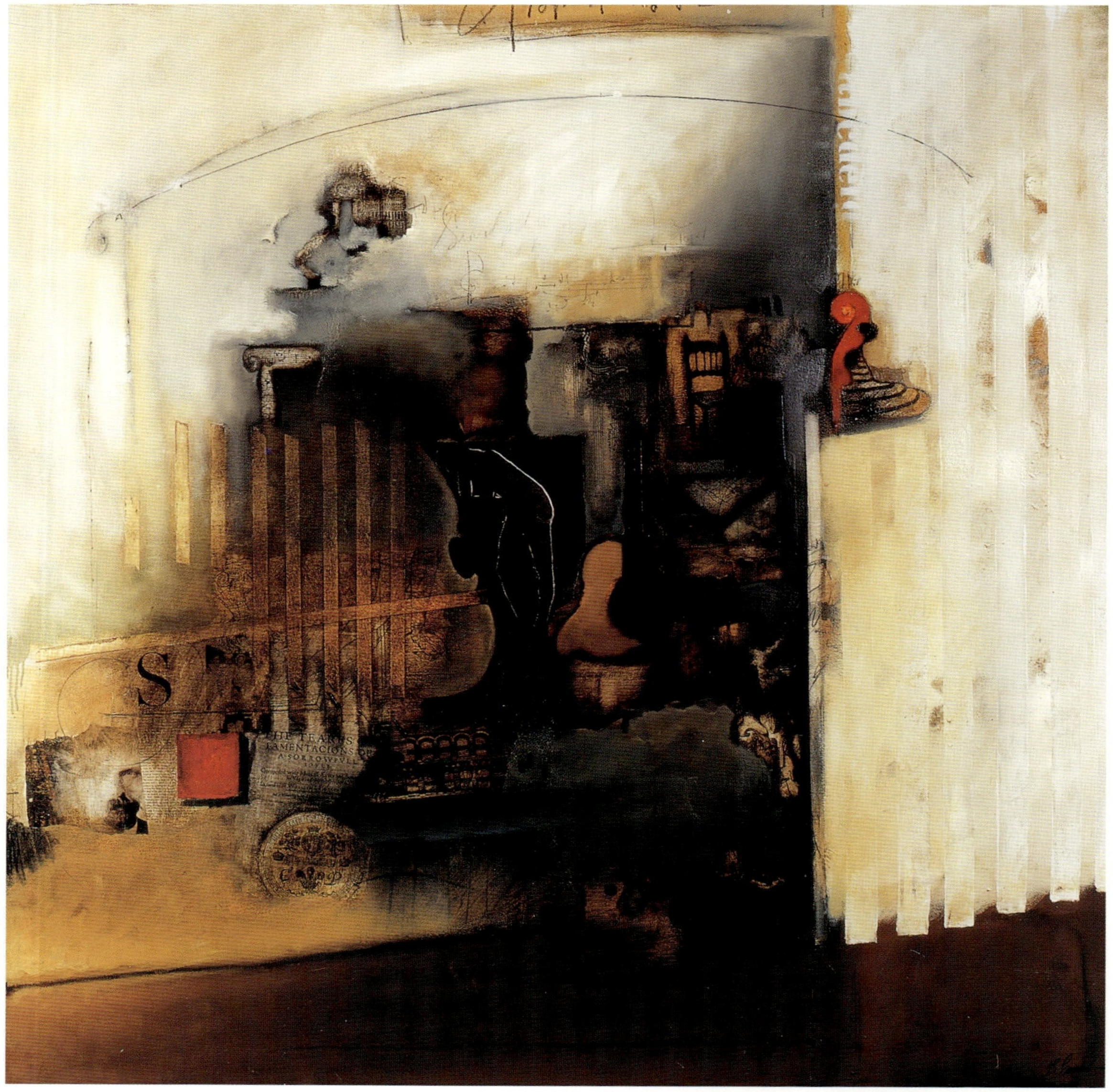

Concerto
Complex Etude I

Mixed Media on Canvas 48"x48"

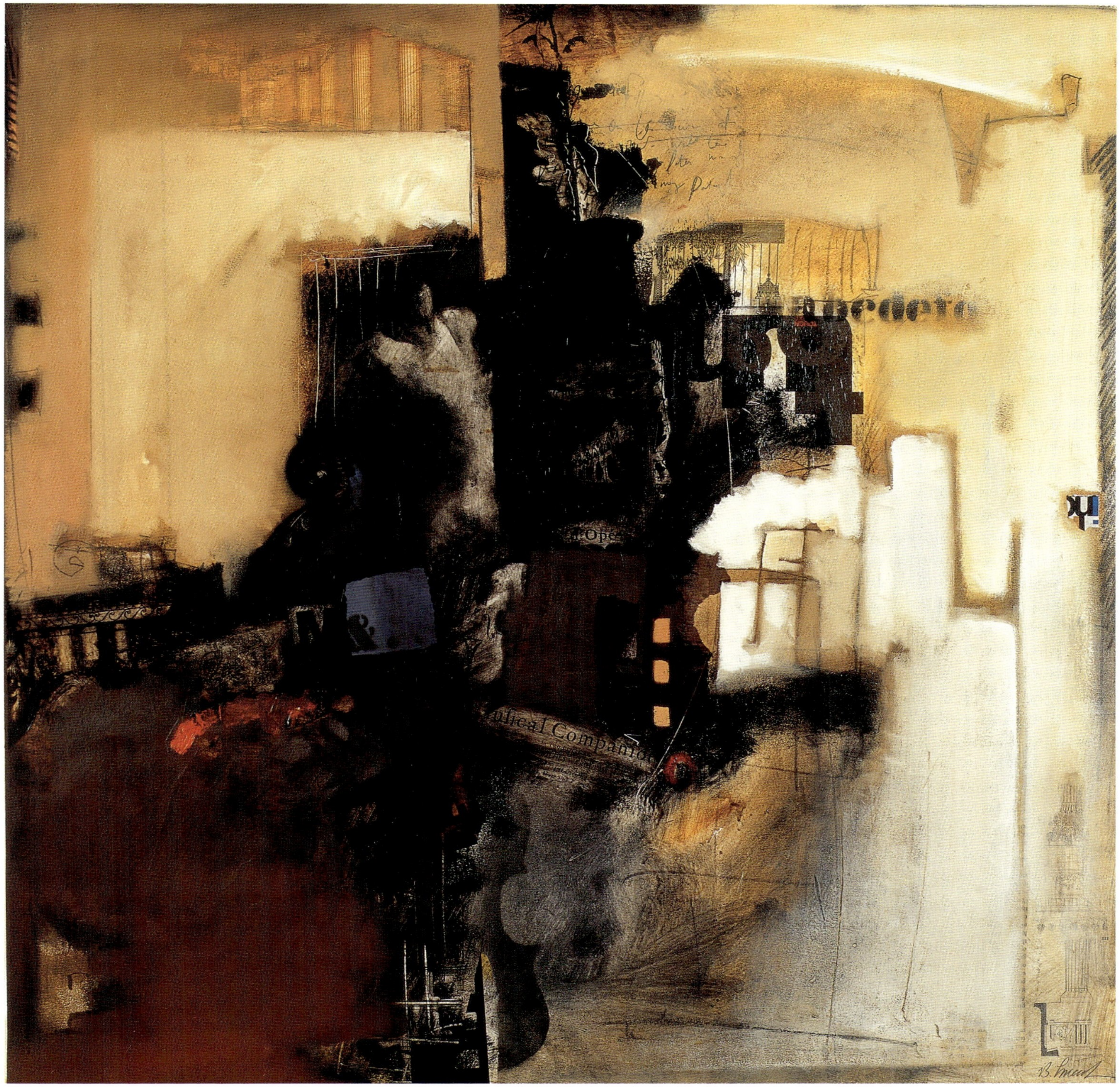

Concerto
Complex Etude II

Mixed Media on Canvas 48"x48"

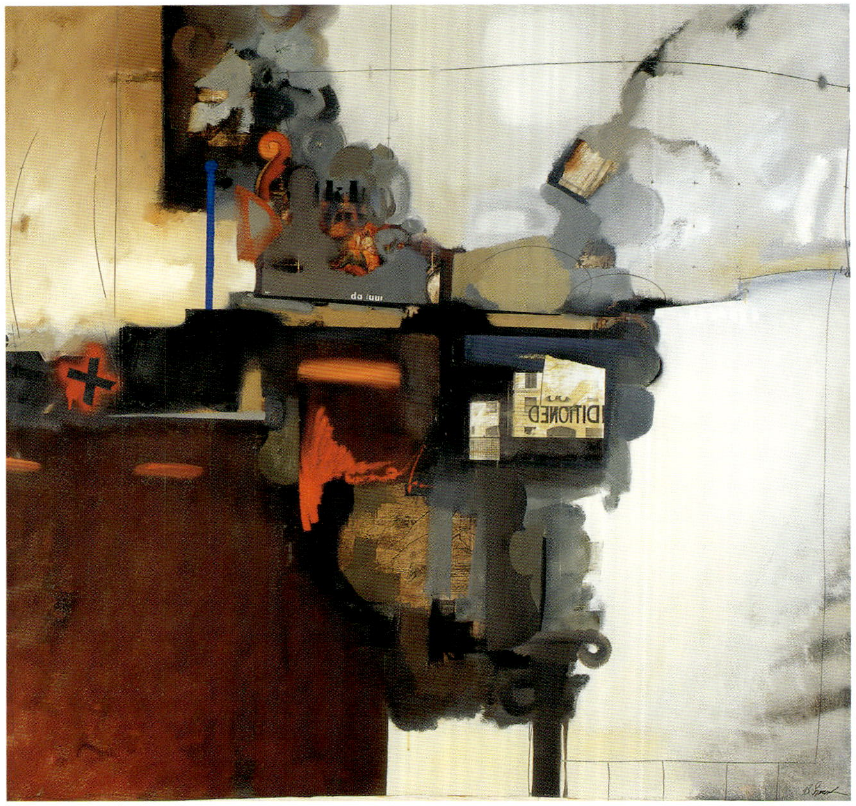

Concerto
Complex Etude III

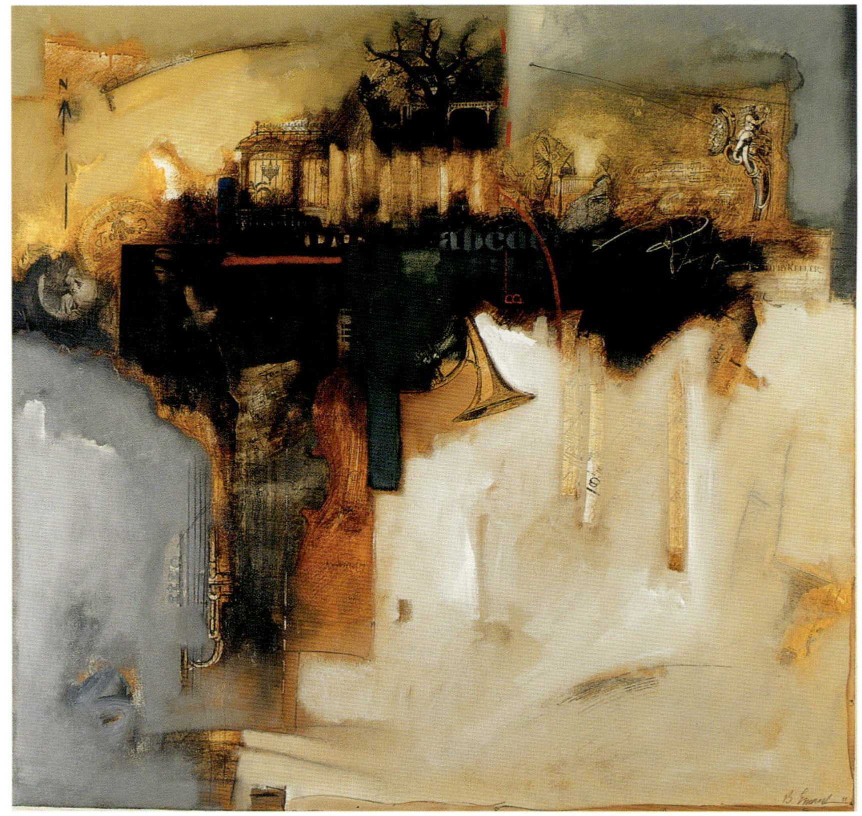

Concerto
Complex Etude IV

Mixed Media on Canvas 48"x48"

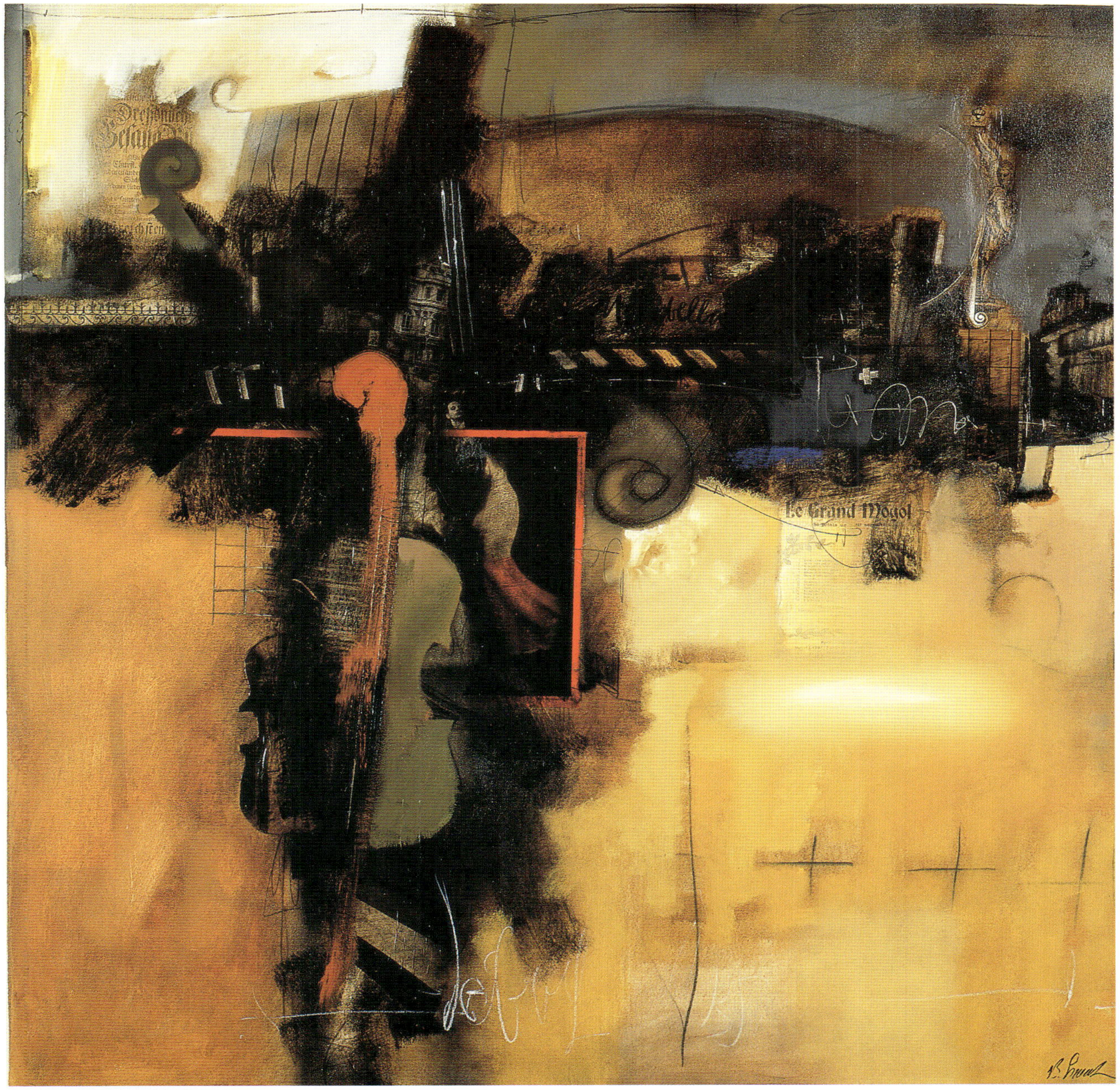

Concerto Complex Etude V

Mixed Media on Canvas 48"x48"

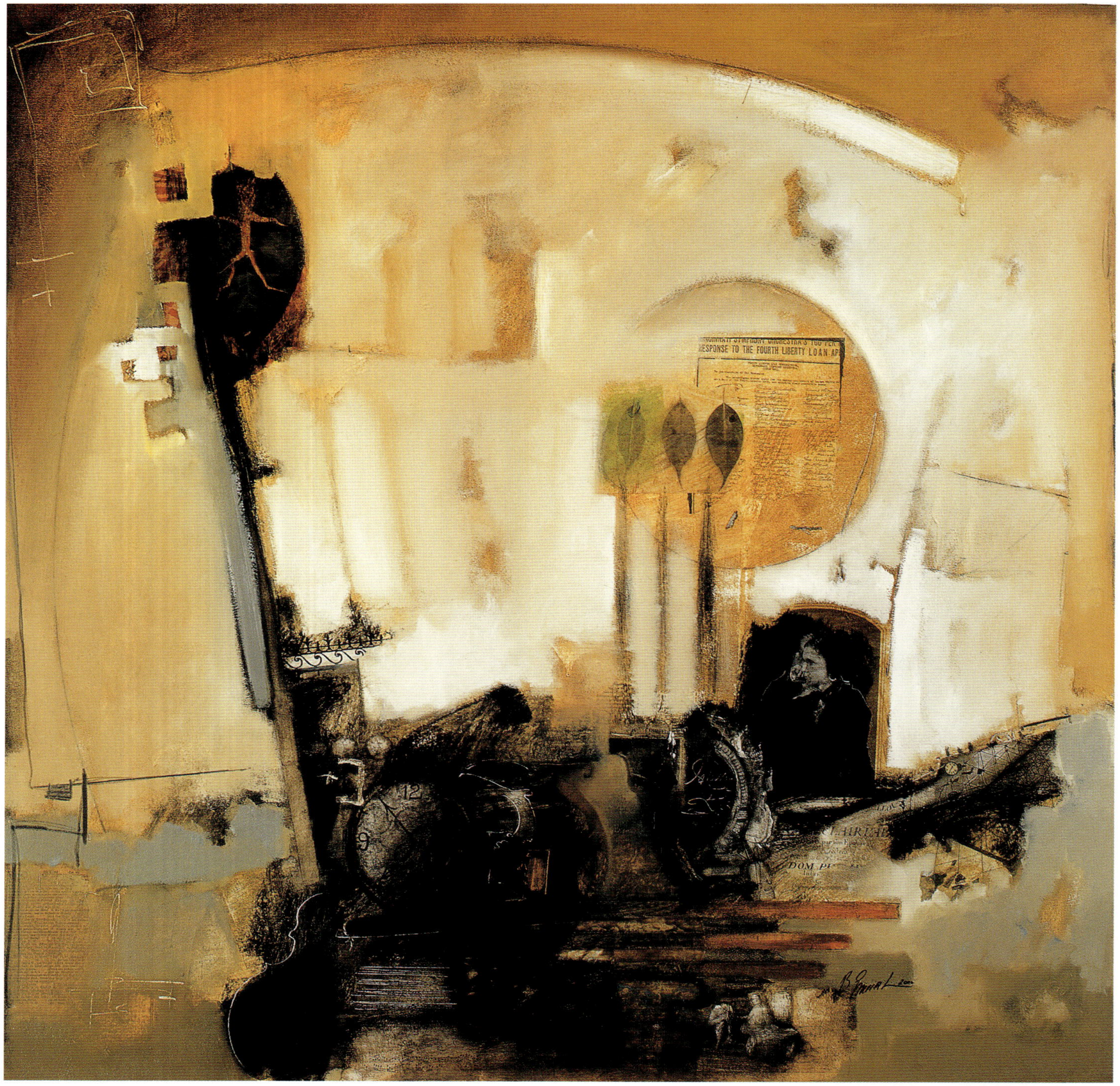

Concerto
Complex Etude VI

 Mixed Media on Canvas 48"x48"

Interview with Emanuel

Interviewer: Abbas Daneshvari, Ph.D.

Are there early influences from your childhood that are present in your contemporary art?

In some regard, the old neighborhoods where I grew up in Shiraz–with their adobe walls and narrow alleyways always opening up to some idyllic landscape–are in my "Hallycon"[6;14-15] series. The moods of "Hallycon" are Iranian and they return to my childhood. I made the paintings pretty much the same way I saw them in my photographs. I consider the beginning of my artistic passion to be in my early photographs of nature back in Iran. All my photos were about the Fall season, a time near the edge of death and rebirth. It is simple, elegant, colorful and full of memory. My photos served as the skeletal structures for my paintings.

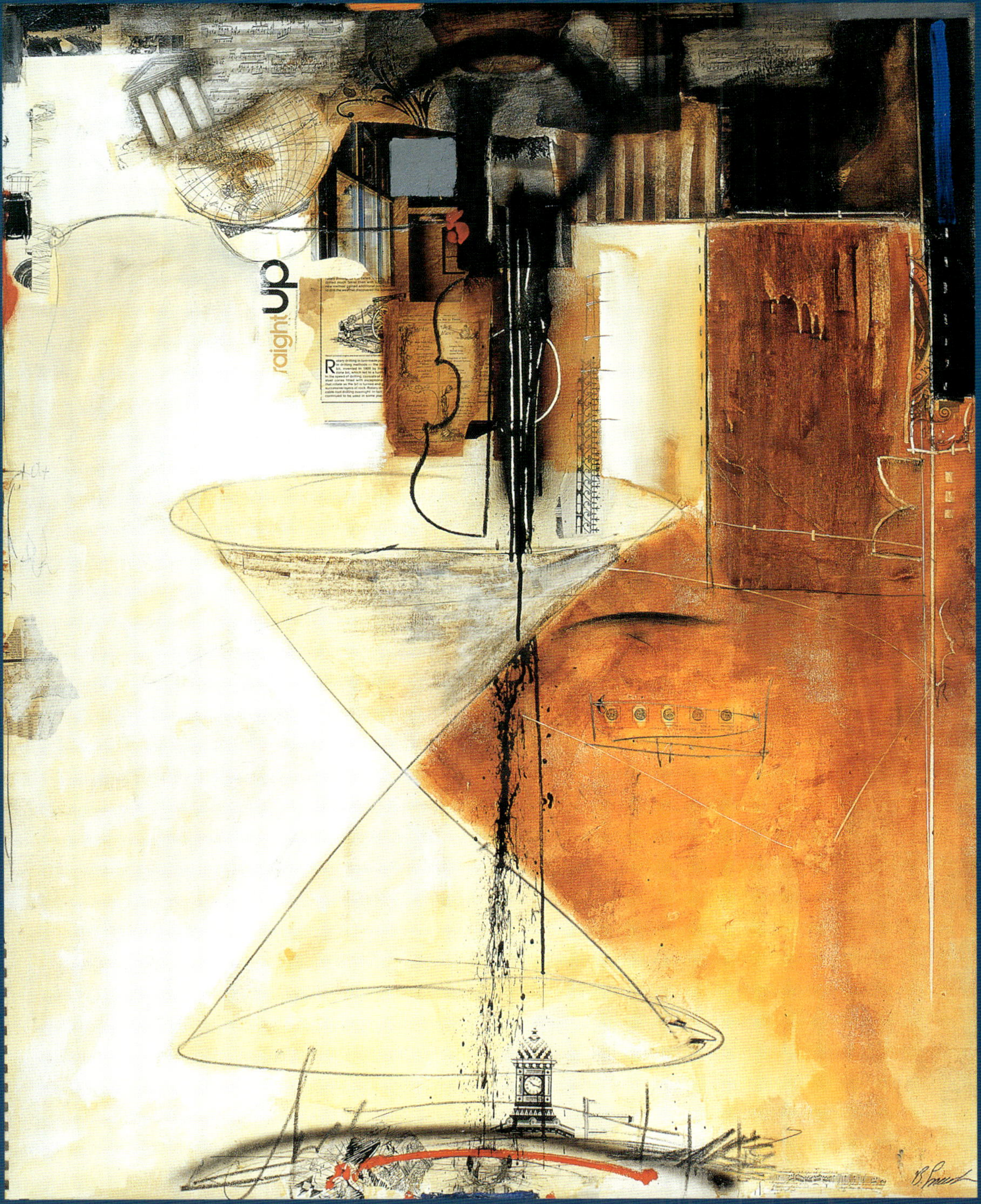

Polyphony

Mixed Media on Canvas 48"x60"

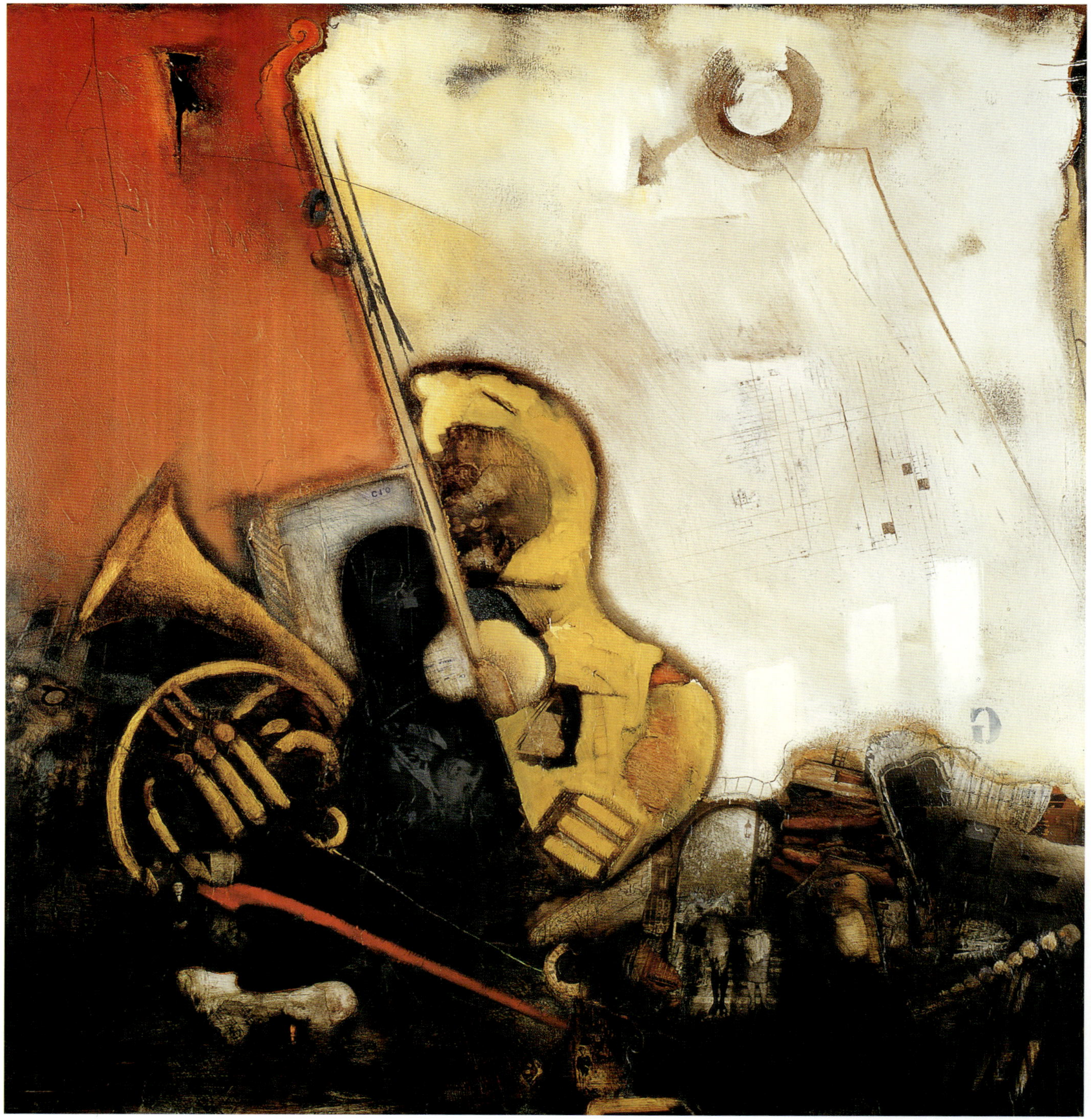

Melodium
Red Rondo II

Mixed Media on Canvas 48"x48"

Silhouette

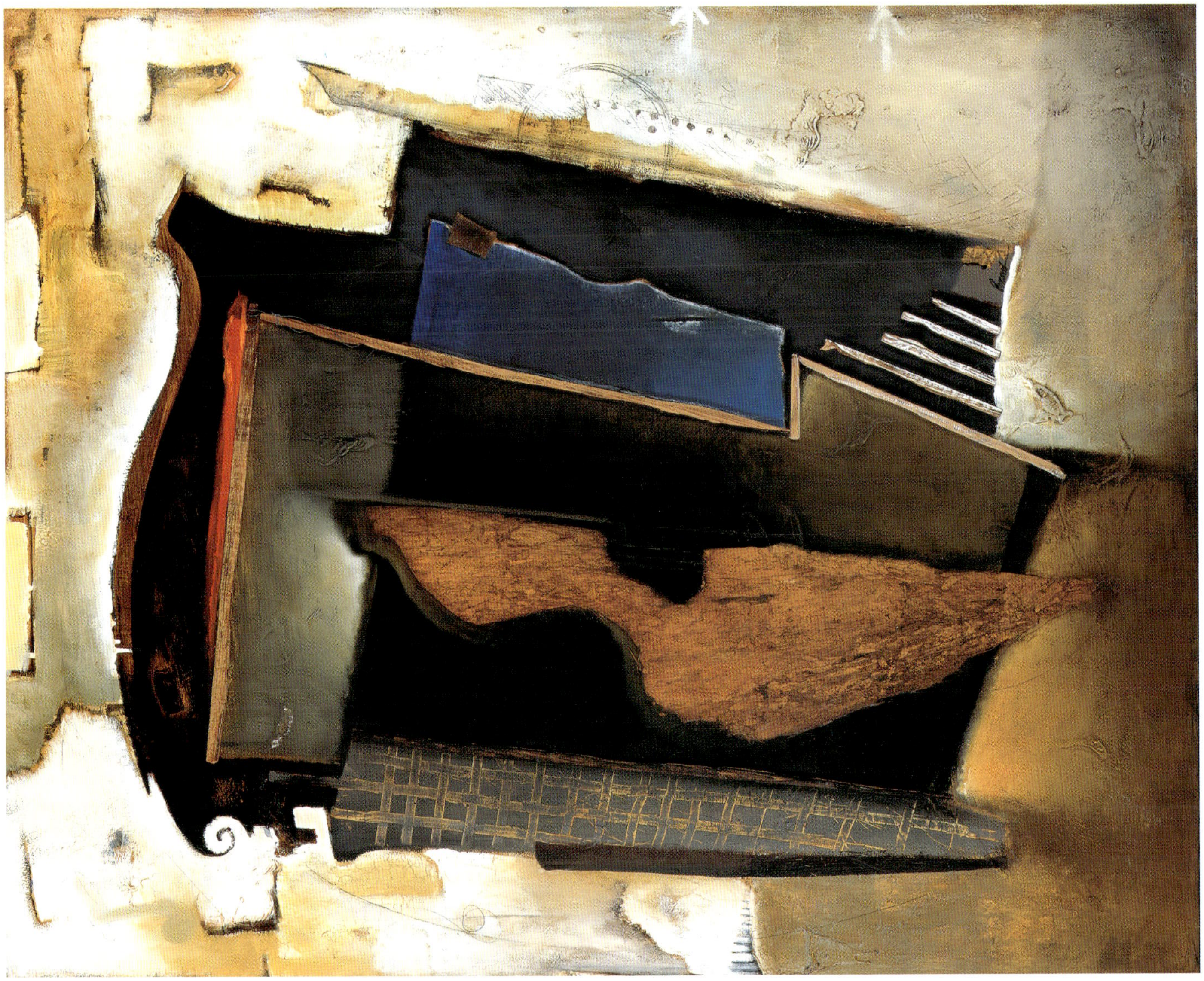

"The world I lived in was another phase, with a different set of priorities and sensations."

How did your obsession for art grow out of your early specialization in mathematics?

The eastern culture rarely encouraged a career in the arts. But art was always my passion. I photographed, drew and painted at every opportunity possible.

What kind of art did you find attractive and emulate when you were in your teens?

The colors and musical shapes of Disney images were fascinating to me. Now that I look back, I realize that these images represented the quintessence of innocence. They also offered a way out of the Persian miniatures.

Why did you seek an alternative to the Persian miniatures?

They were not me. Persian miniatures represented one phase of Iranian art and life. The world I lived in was another phase, with a different set of priorities and sensations. We were no longer purely Persian—or anything else. In the late twentieth century the world had become smaller and like a kind of artistic melting pot. So, the established traditions of our distinct histories were quickly becoming obsolete.

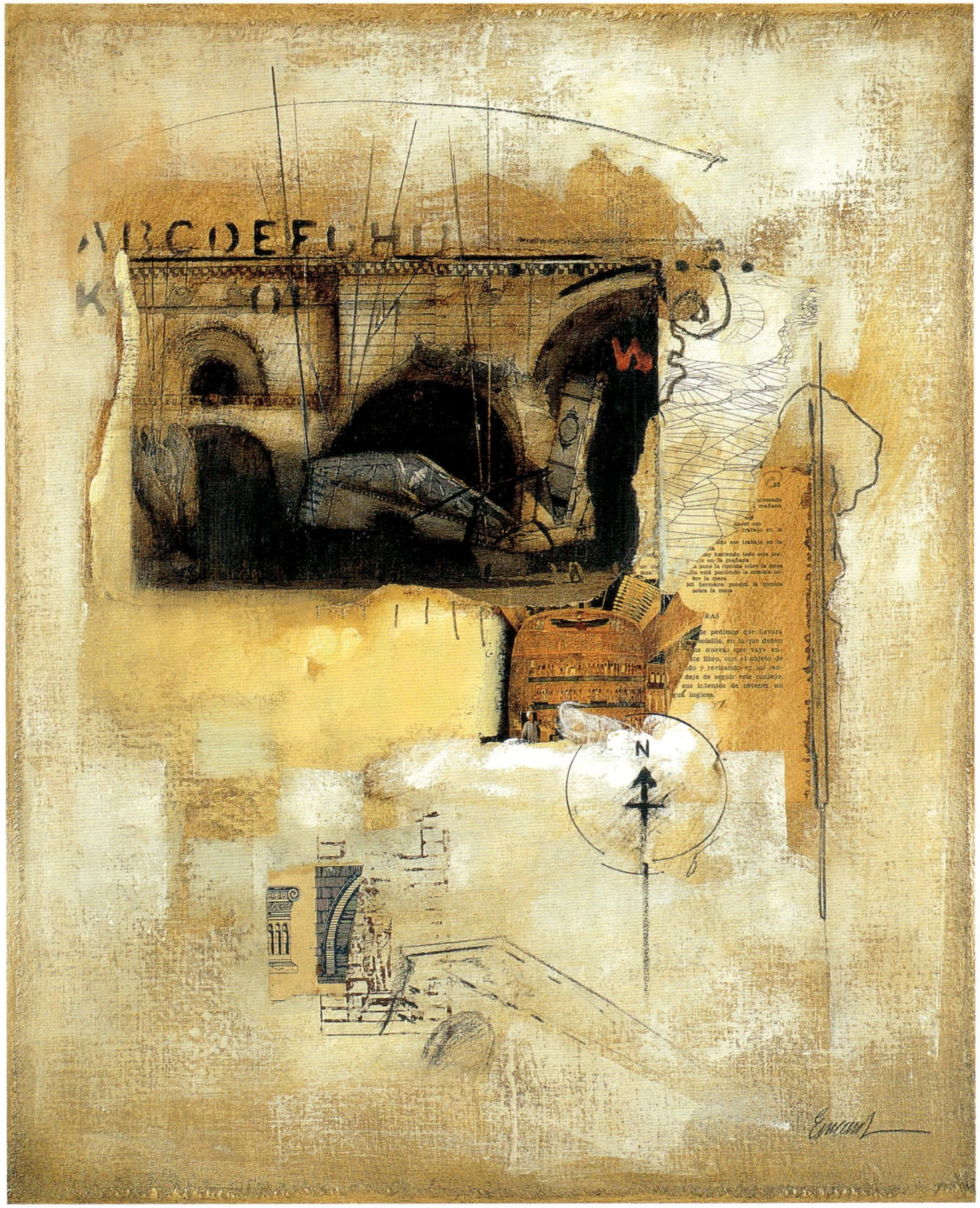

Passages
Memorabilia I

Mixed Media on Paper 18"x24"

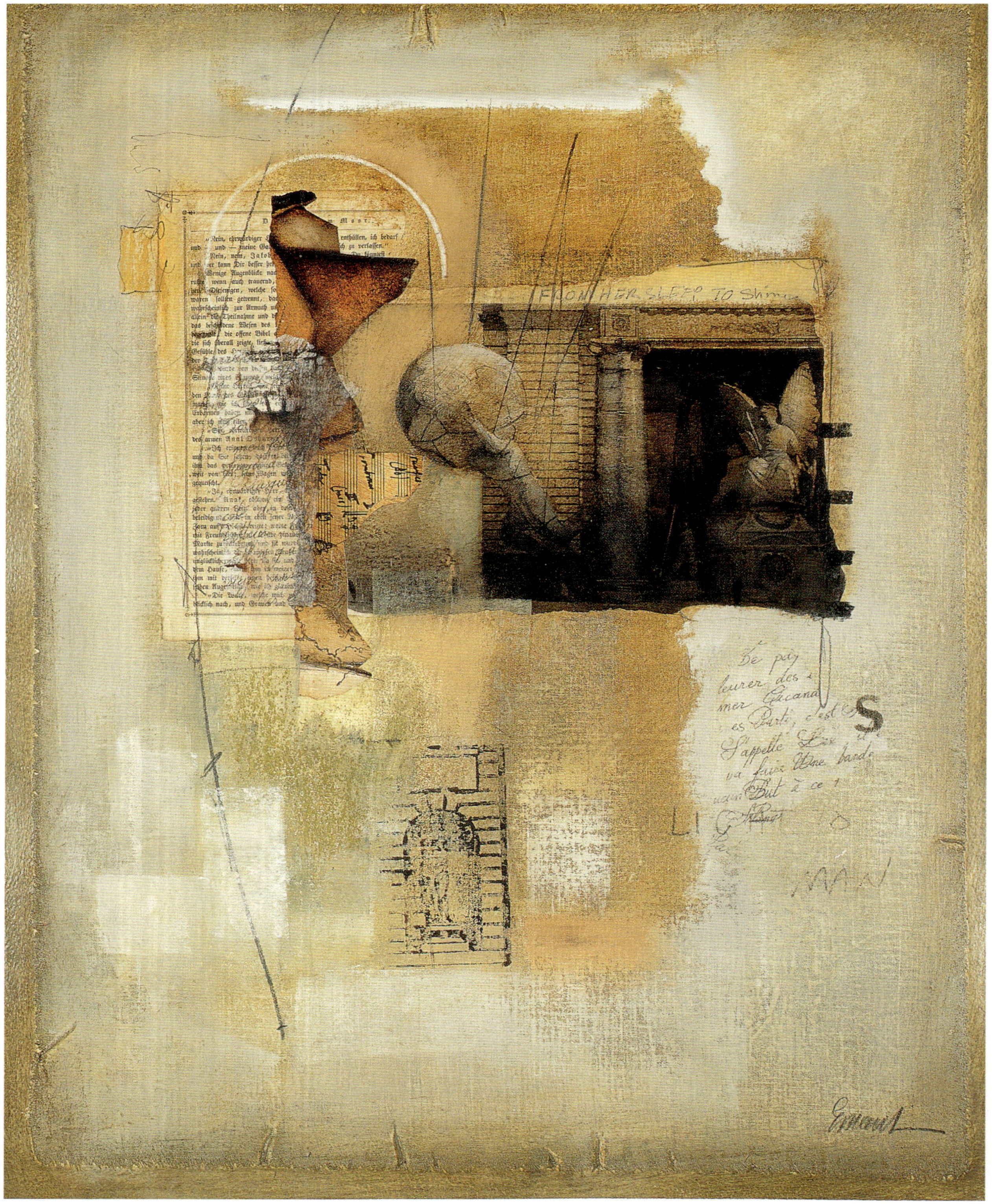

Passages Memorabilia II

Mixed Media on Paper 18"x24"

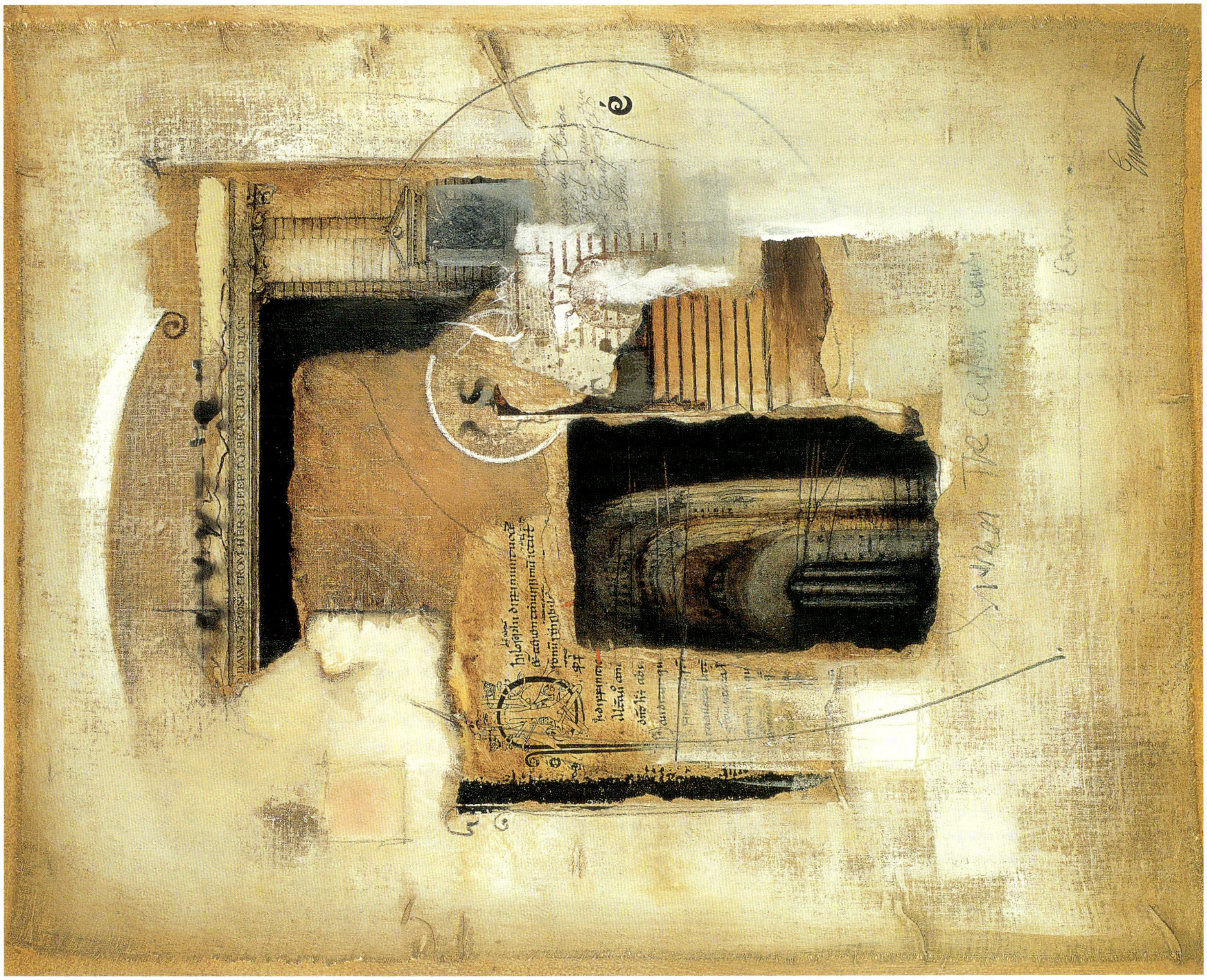

Passages
Memorabilia III

"The profound changes caused by migration also liberated my soul and allowed me to pursue my heart's desires."

When did your career in the arts actually begin?

Art as my life – that is how I like to phrase it – began after I arrived in the States in 1987. The profound changes caused by migration also liberated my soul and allowed me to pursue my heart's desires.

Was migration difficult?

Yes, I had to remind myself of the hundreds and perhaps thousands who had immigrated to the States in the wake of World War II and after – including DeKooning, Gorky and many other artists like them. Immigration proved harder for some than for others. Without getting too detailed, I will simply say that it is not easy to escape political and cultural uncertainty. Even though I wasn't personally traumatized, it was not easy.

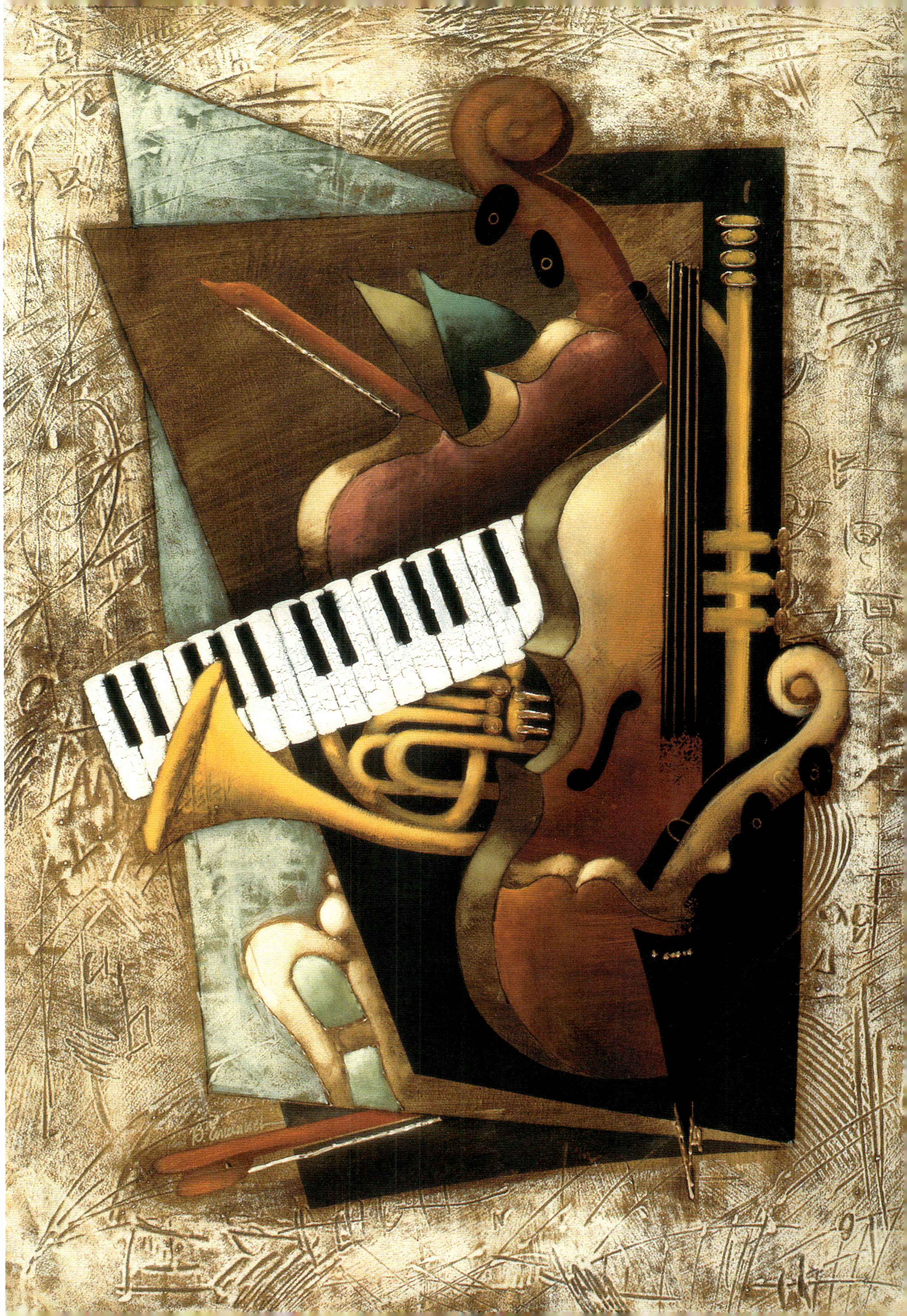

Orchestration II

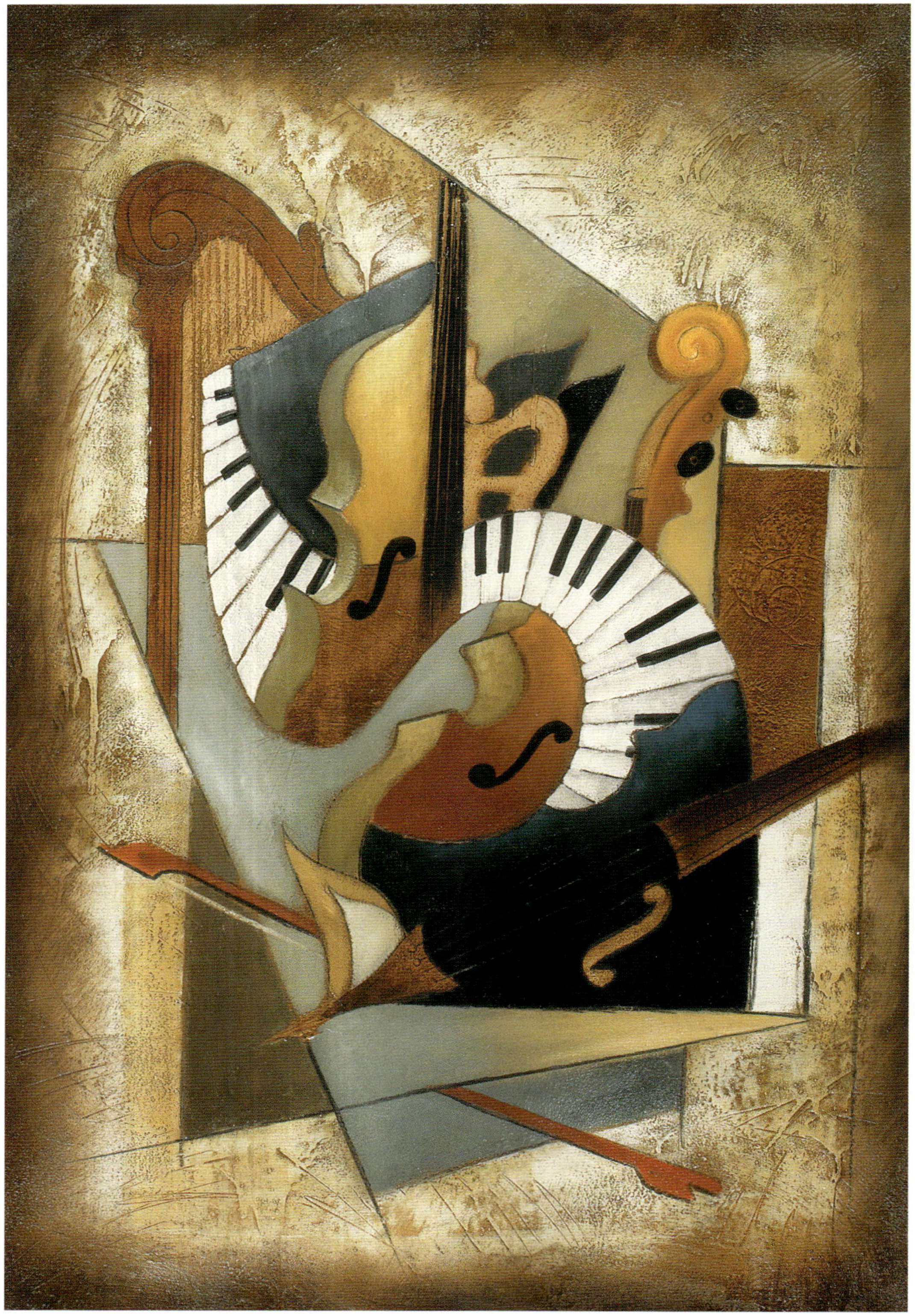

"My life began to have an emotional and spiritual focus again and painting was making it possible."

Orchestration V

Mixed Media on Paper 30"x44"

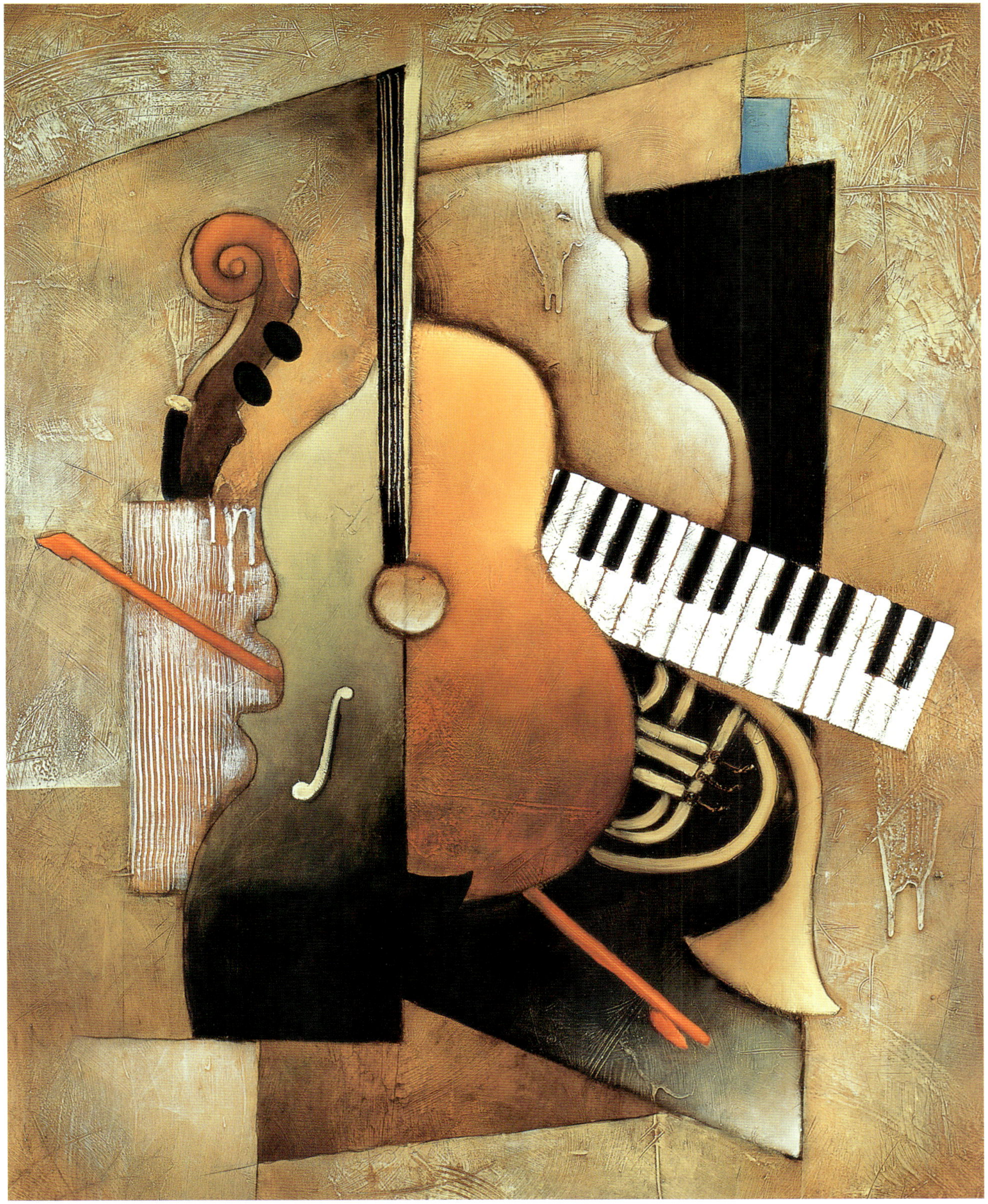

Orchestration XIV

Mixed Media on Paper 30"x44"

Once in the States, what was the spark that ignited your passion in the arts?

Without question, seeing art that I felt was partly or mostly one with me. My life began to have an emotional and spiritual focus again and painting was making it possible. Through art I had found myself. All of this became possible when I started to study in Atlanta. One thing led to another and here I am.

Do you recall a first encounter with a certain artwork that moved you emotionally and propelled you to become an artist?

Yes, of course. It was Motherwell's "Elegy" paintings. His paintings combined the innocence of children and the expertise of masters in a seamless way. He offered me, through his understanding of color and his bold use of black, a wholly different way of looking at nature. He always wanted to return to a pristine source of creativity and sometimes that meant to start all over again from scratch. But you can imagine how few people in the middle eastern culture understood my early fascination with an abstract painter like Motherwell.

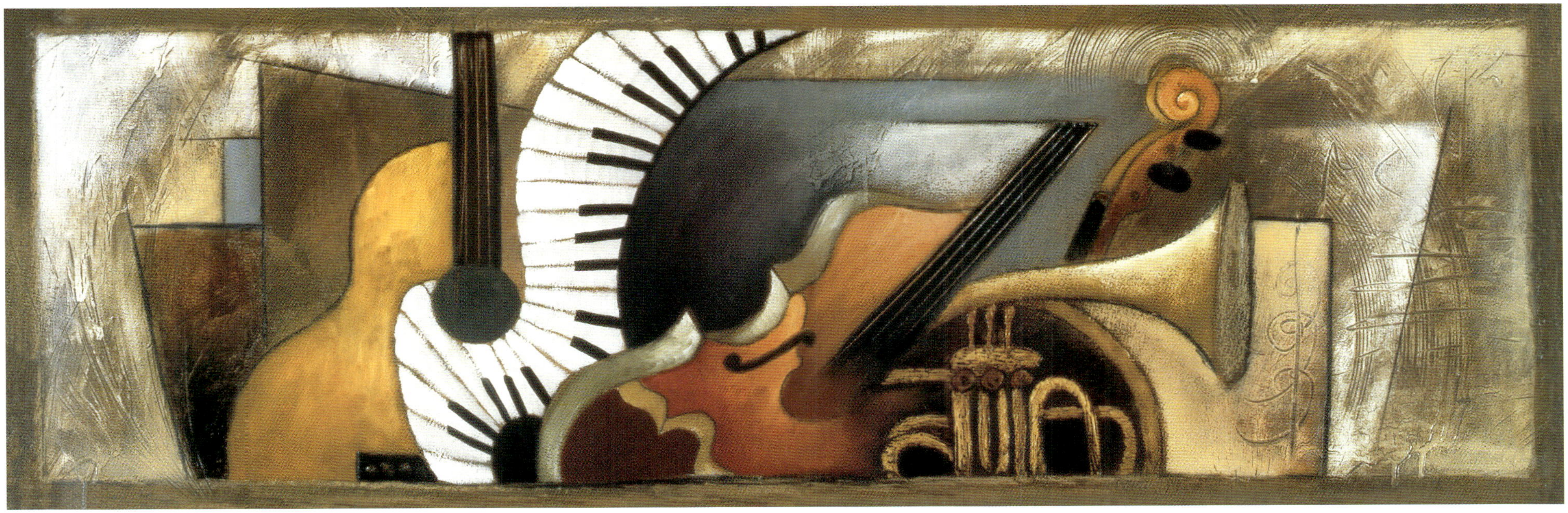

Orchestration IV

Mixed Media on Paper 54"x19"

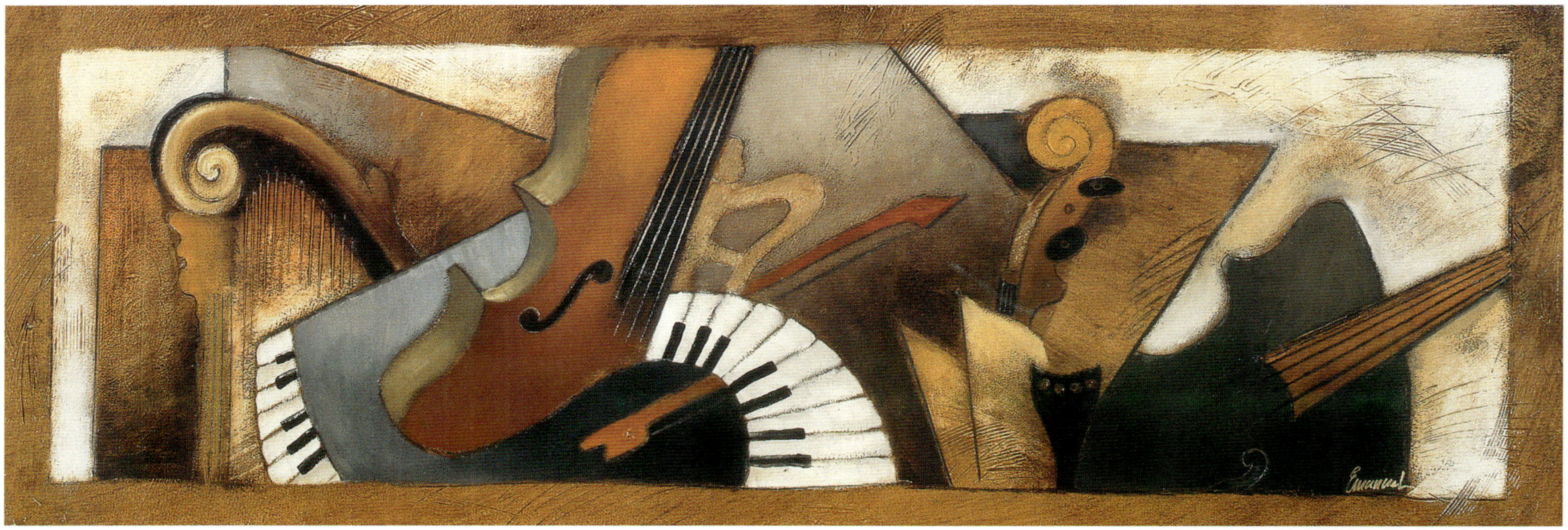

Orchestration XII

Mixed Media on Paper 54"x19"

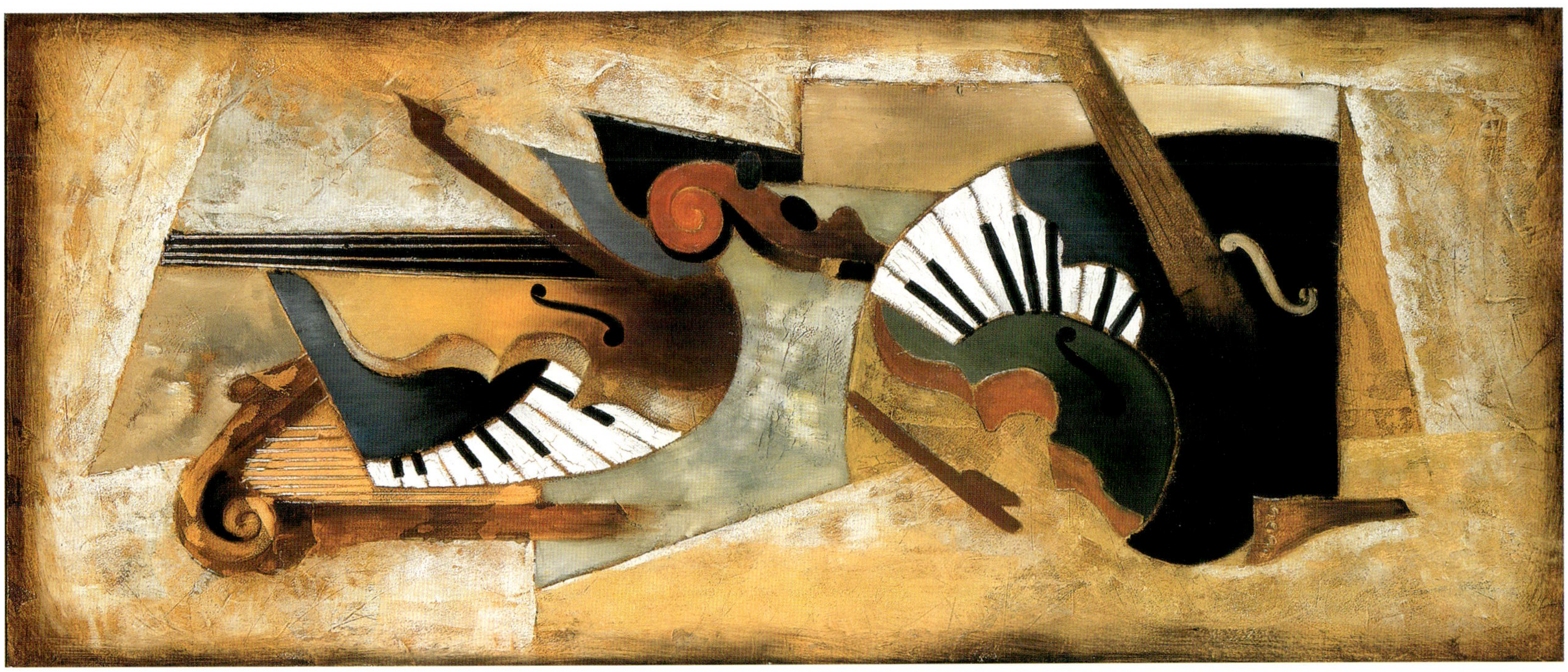

Orchestration XI

"The closer a painting is
to the heart, the more
musical it becomes."

Yet, Motherwell has profound affinities to oriental art.
Do you see any relation between the two?

In retrospect, I recognize how the mysticism of the Orient and the individuation of the Occident are to some degree one and the same. Kandinsky and Malevich, among many others, are examples of artists who have defined Modernism as a conflation of mysticism and individuation. But it was Motherwell's bold gestures that deeply moved me on a physical level. He seemed free and unconstrained. His movements were musical symphonies.

Music and musical instruments are obviously an inextricable part of your paintings.
What do they signify?

When I paint, I not only feel music; I feel that I am a song. I am part of the rhythmic flow thrown into the river of time. Music guides my moves, for it reaches beyond language and consciousness. I – like MacDonald Wright and Delaunay who wanted to transform their paintings into musical expressions – also seek the open, silent spaces of art. The closer a painting is to the heart, the more musical it becomes. I look for honesty in my expressions and music has always been an ally of mine.

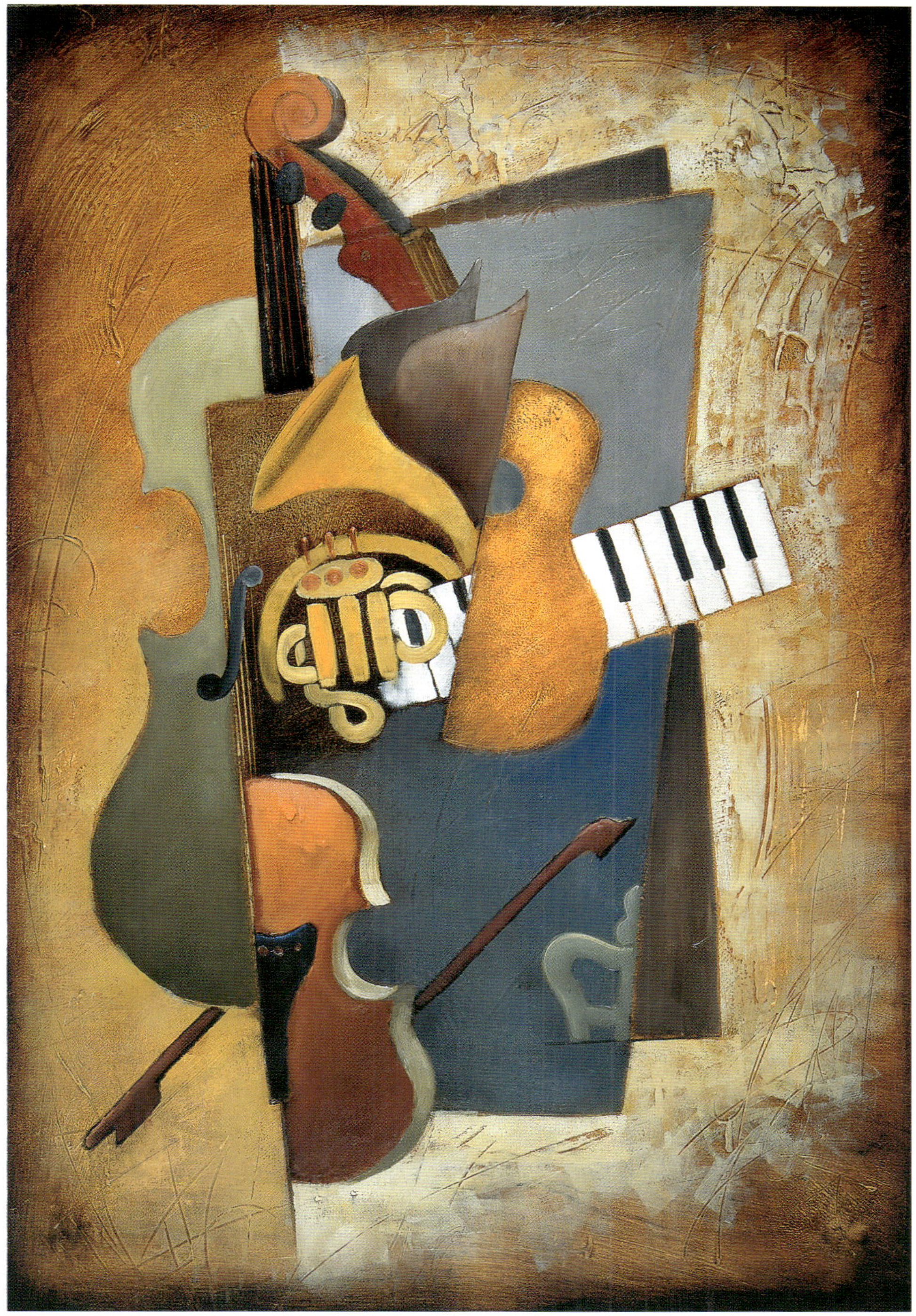

Orchestration
Musica Profundis I

Mixed Media on Paper
30"x44"

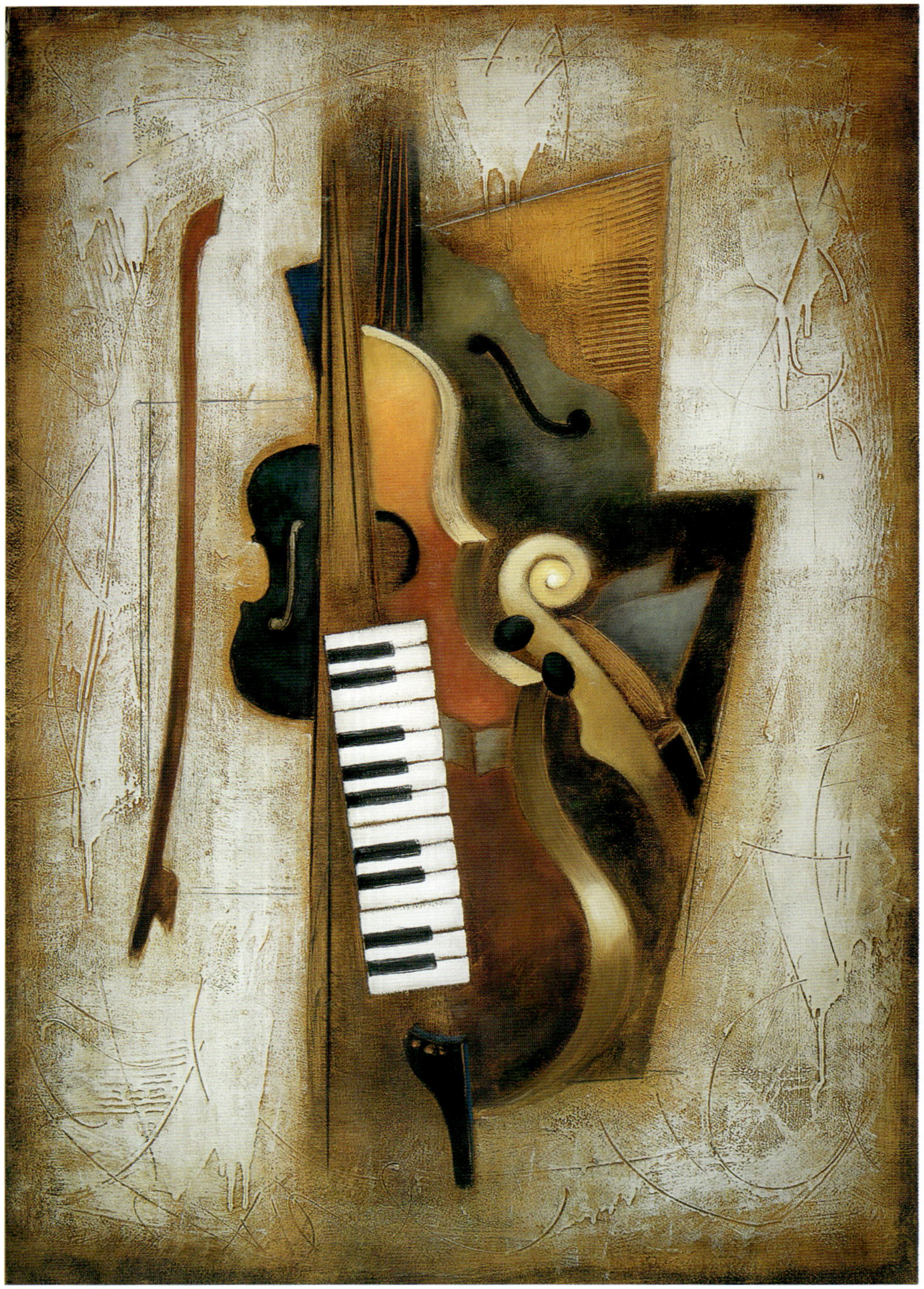

Orchestration
Musica Profundis II

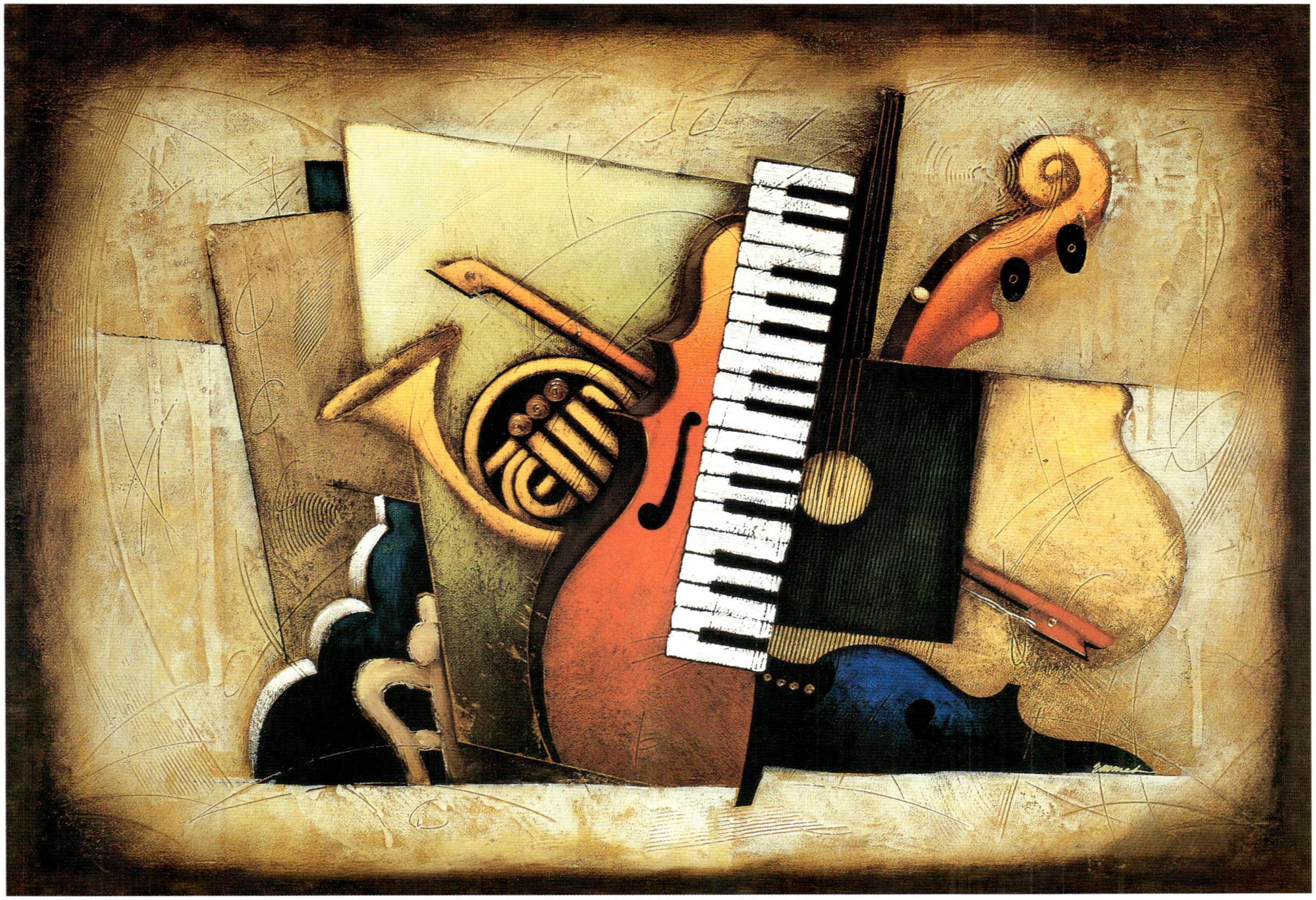

"Rauschenberg taught me how to move from the image to abstraction, preserving both and also destroying them."

Orchestration
Musica Profundis III

How would you describe your allusions to Renaissance and Roman art?

What I love most about the Renaissance is its virtuosity of representation. A Renaissance painting is like a Paganini composition; it is difficult to write and you have to be doubly virtuous to play it. Technically, my paintings allude to both the Renaissance and Baroque. These techniques age the imagery and evoke a sense of dreaminess about them.

Whom else do you admire among the western modern masters?

Aside from Motherwell, MacDonald Wright and Delauney, I also love Rauschenberg and Tapis. Rauschenberg taught me how to move from the image to abstraction, preserving both and also destroying them. Rauschenberg does not have the bold and daring gestures of Motherwell, but he certainly knows how to balance the contrasting currents of art.

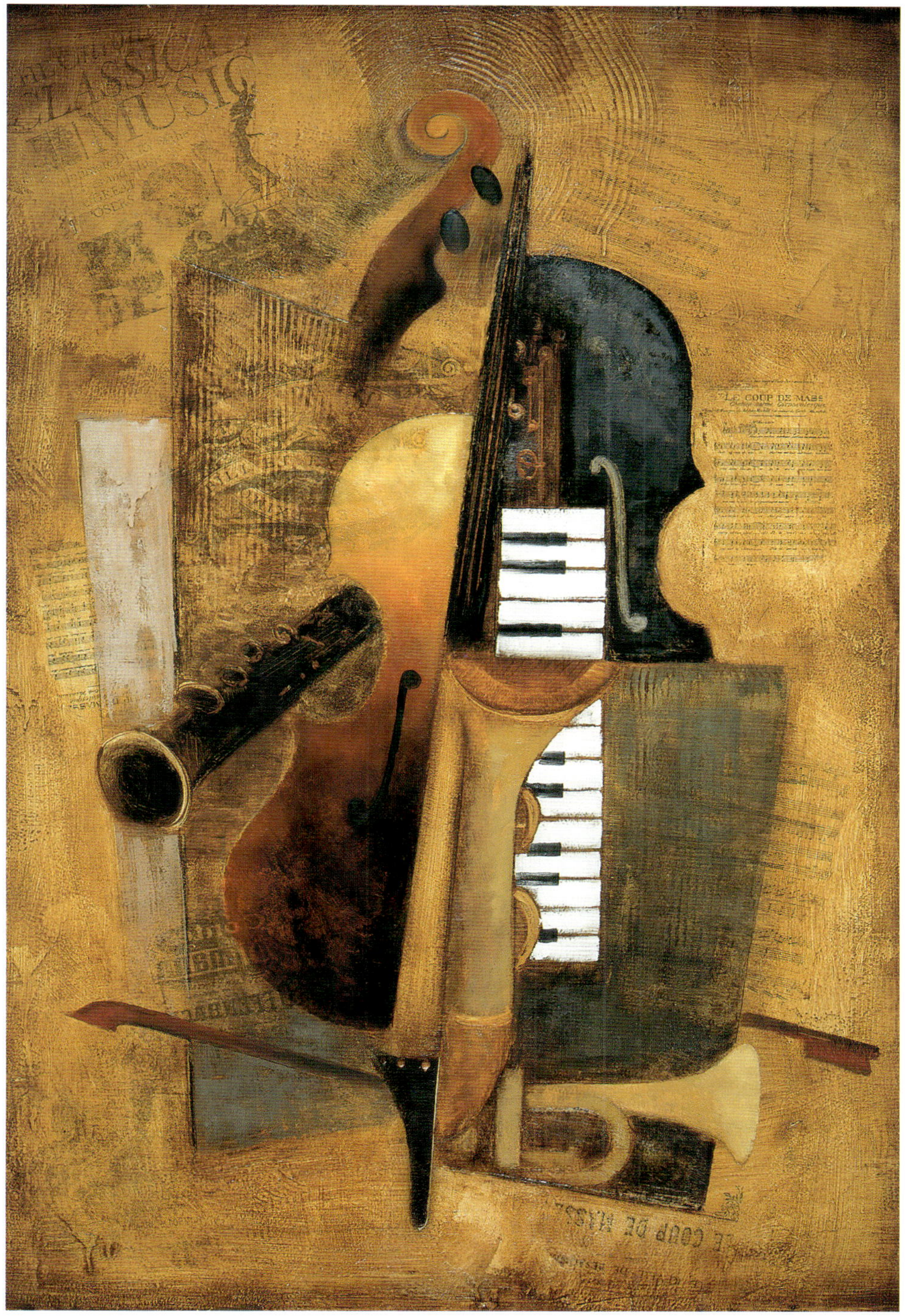

Orchestration
Musica Profundis IV

Mixed Media on Paper
30"x44"

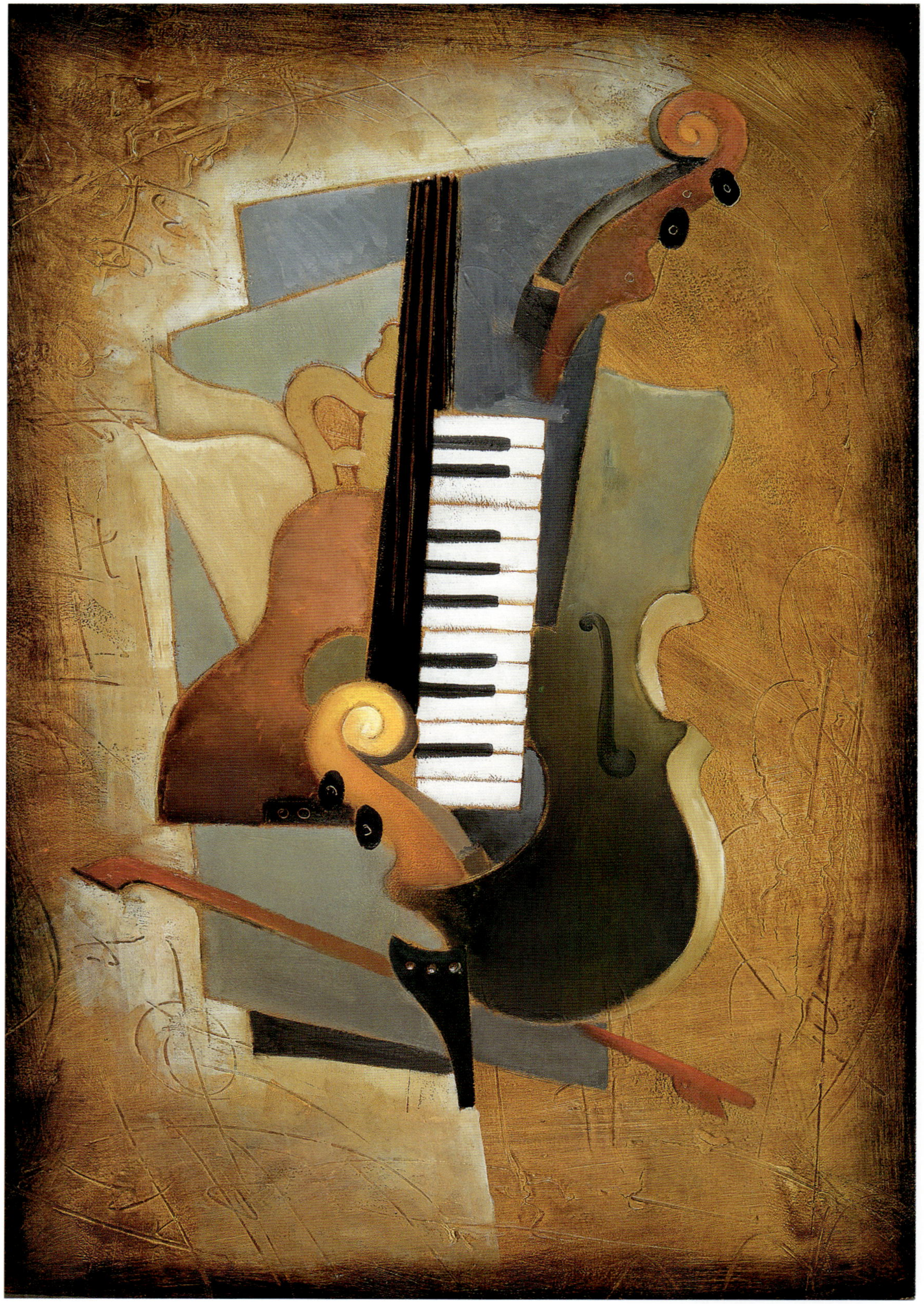

Orchestration
Musica Profundis V

Mixed Media on Paper 30"x44"

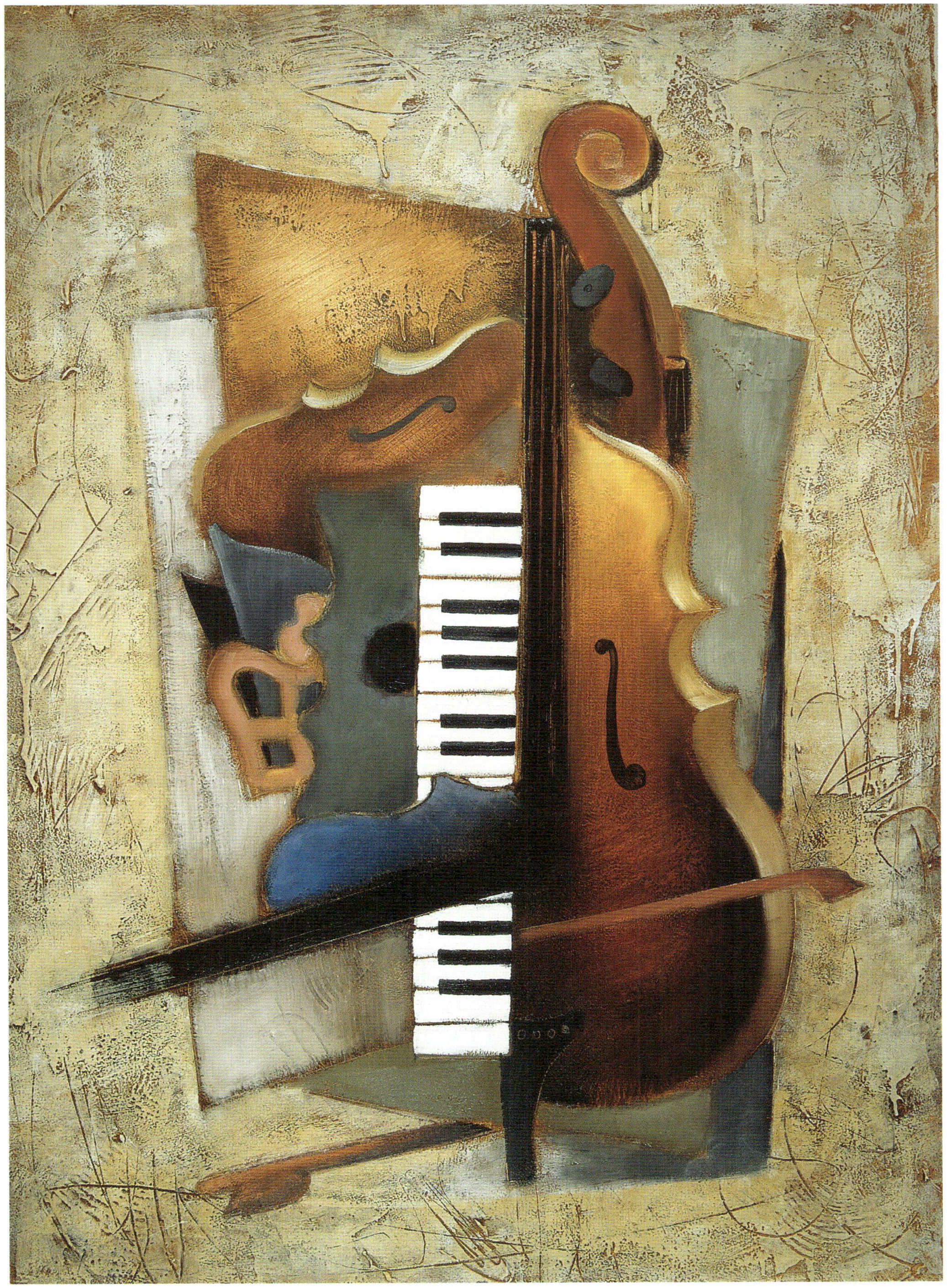

"I manage to find release from the object and the objective world through the fragmentations and assimilations of collage."

Orchestration
Musica Profundis VI

Mixed Media on Paper 30"x44"

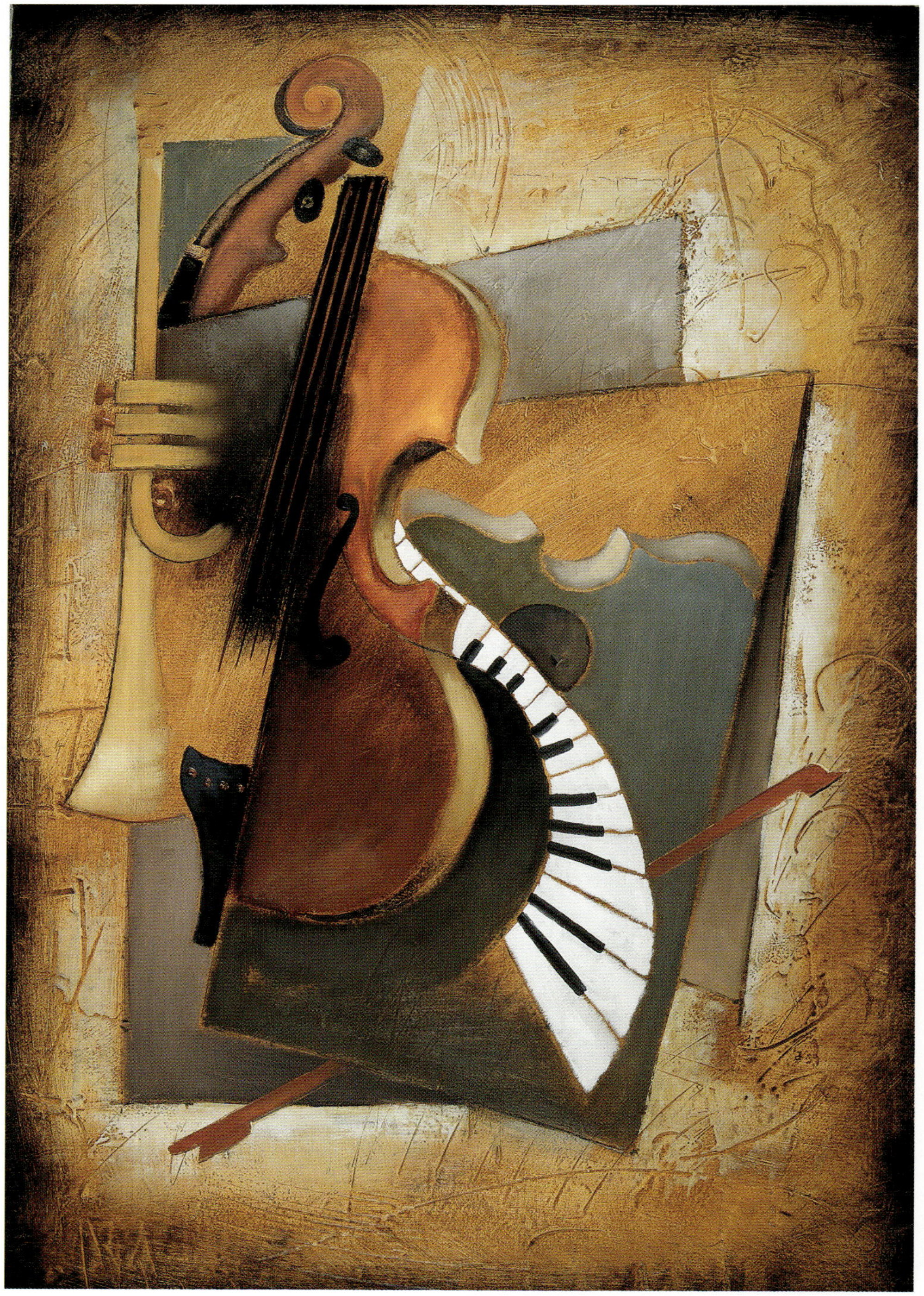

Orchestration
Orchestra Aura I

Mixed Media on Paper 30"x44"

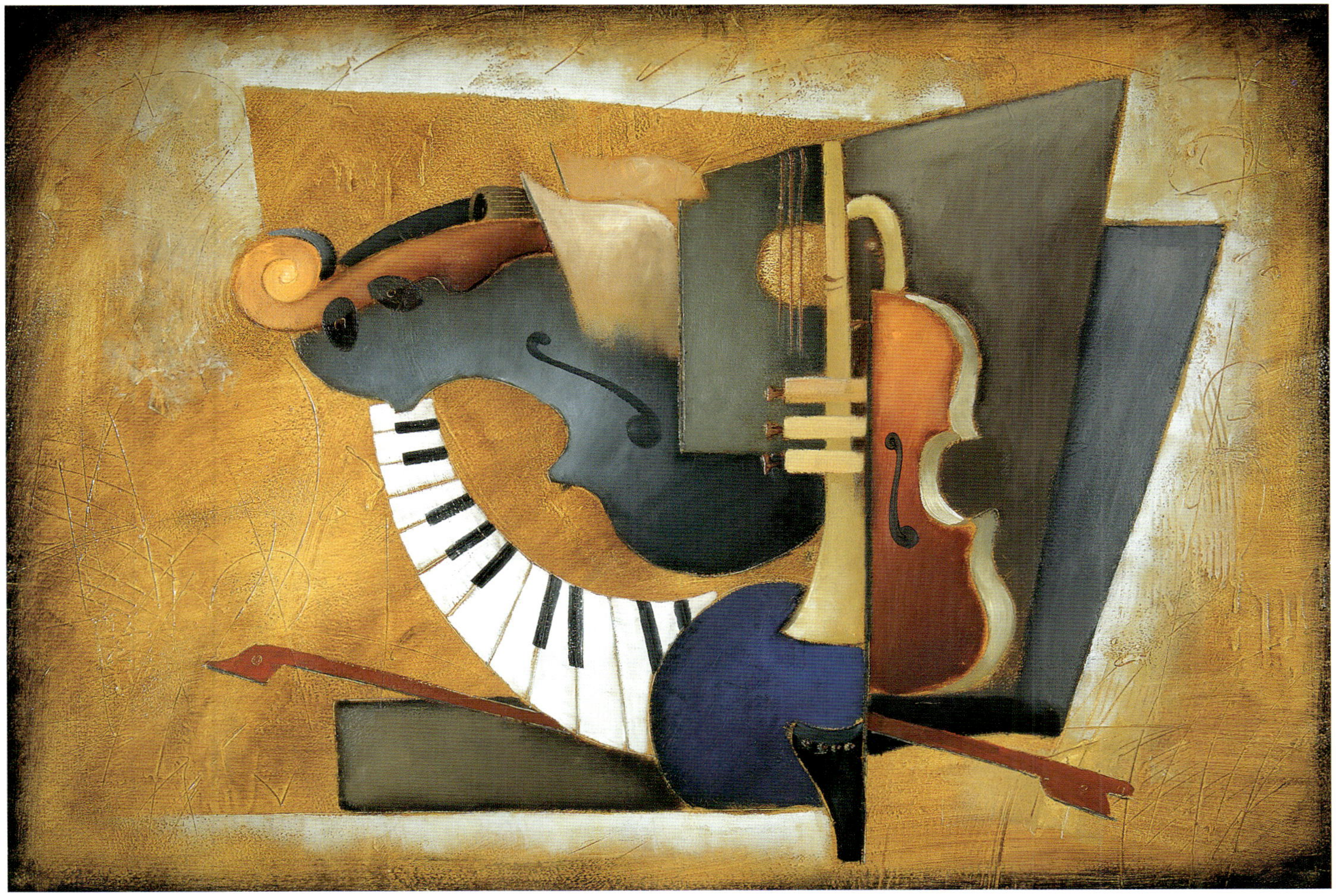

Orchestration
Orchestra Aura II

Mixed Media on Paper 44"x30"

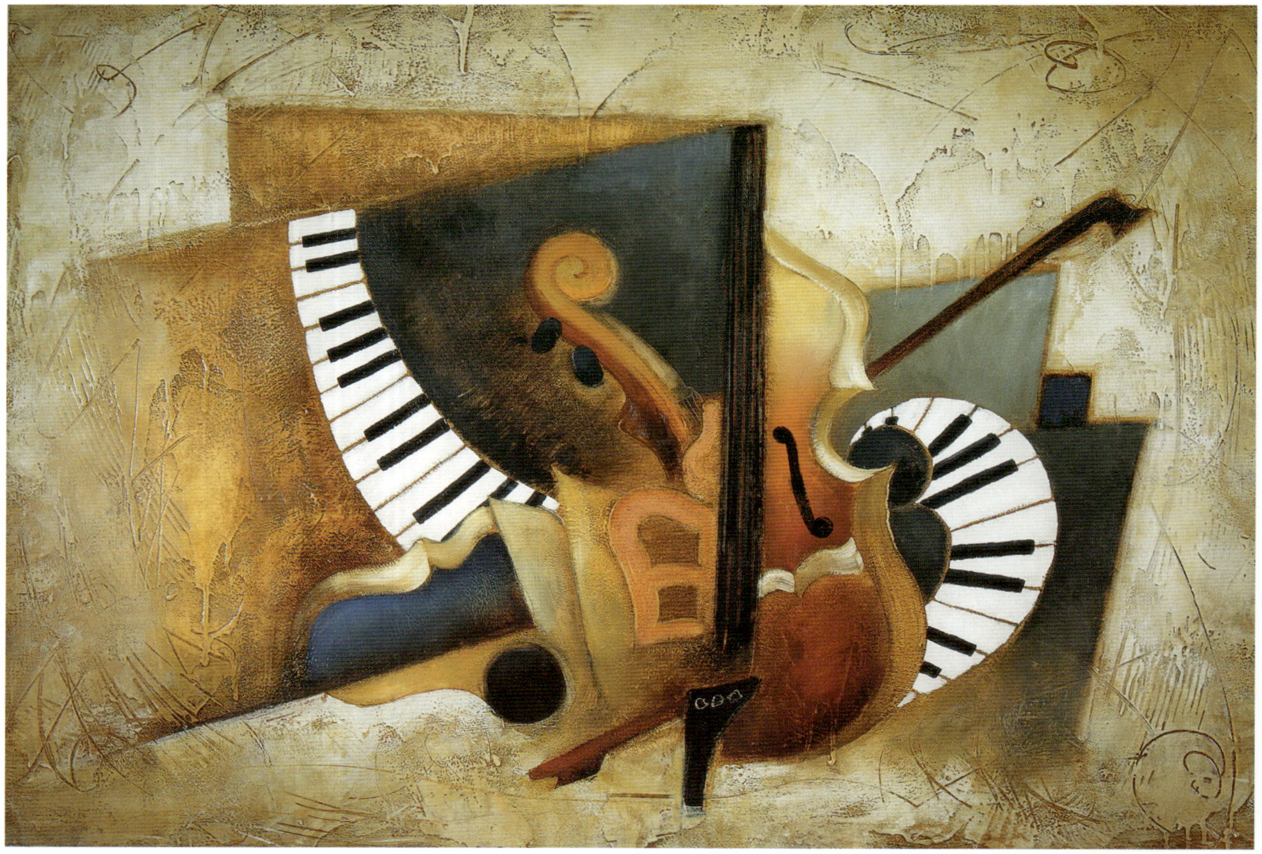

How did the technique of collage start to appear in your works?

Collage, for me, is a way of abstracting even the ordinary and the most familiar of items. I manage to find release from the object and the objective world through the fragmentation and assimilation of collage. At the same time, something of the object's uniqueness remains and survives even while it is decontextualized. Rauschenberg uses mixed media in a manner that transports me from reality to something else. I also love Braque; I think more of him than I do of Picasso. It is the way Braque mixes bits of life and makes a new transcendent vision of them. Most importantly, the use of words excites me. In this regard, I think I have merged something of the Persian calligraphic paintings with the European collage. It is therefore doubly meaningful to me.

Orchestration
Orchestra Aura III

44"x30"

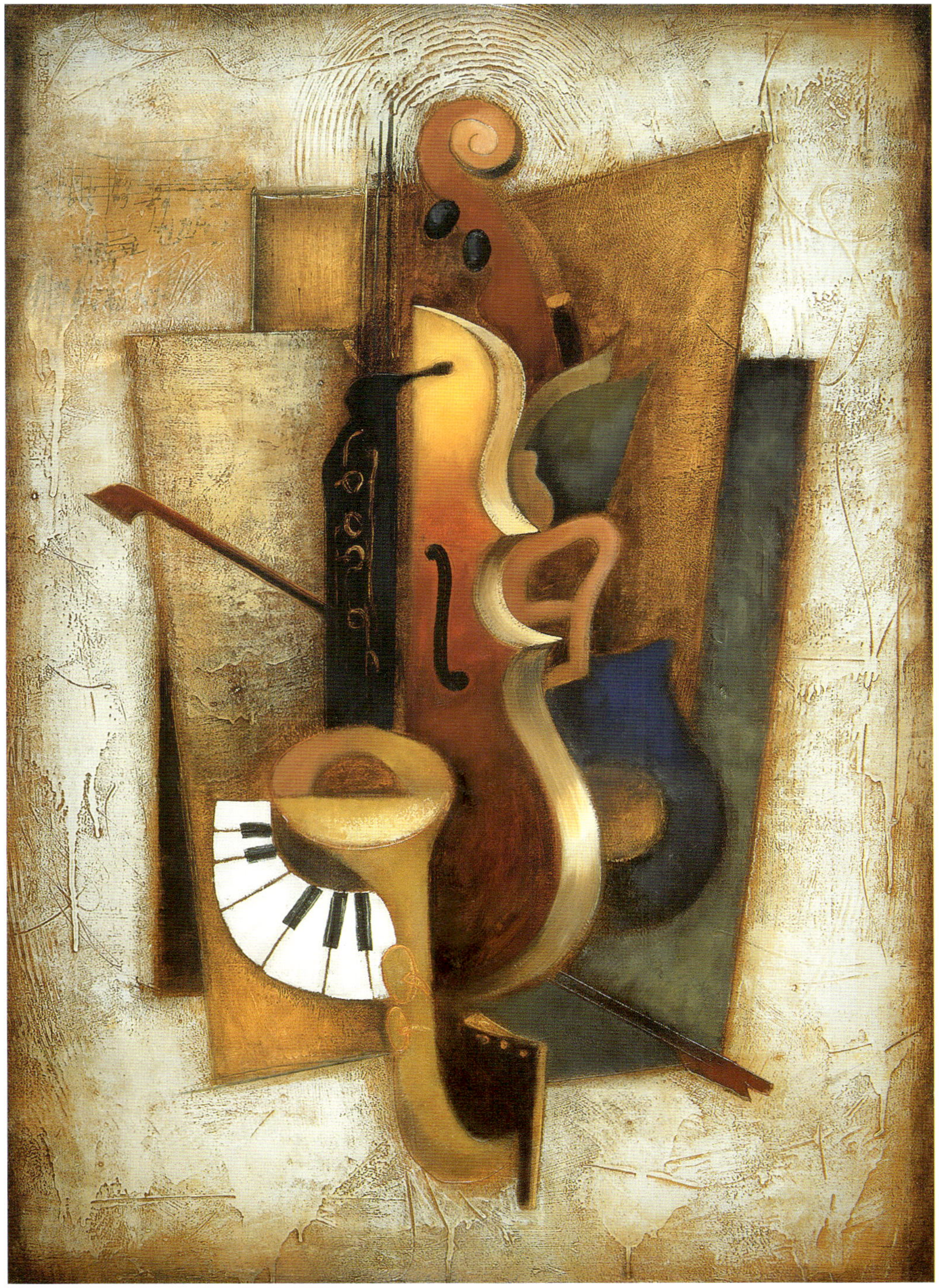

Orchestration
Orchestra Aura IV

Mixed Media on Paper 30"x44"

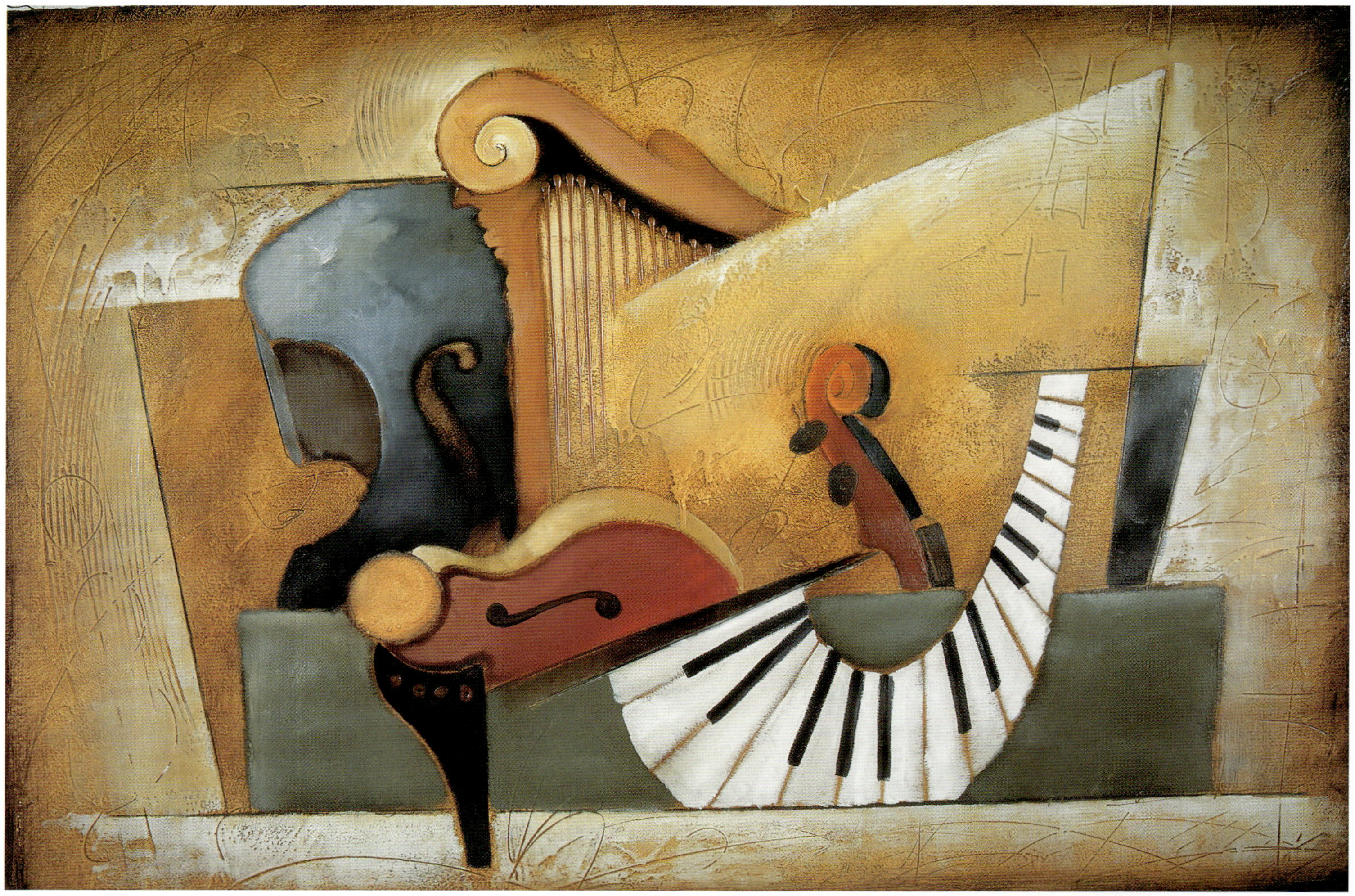

Orchestration
Orchestra Aura V

Mixed Media on Paper 44"x30"

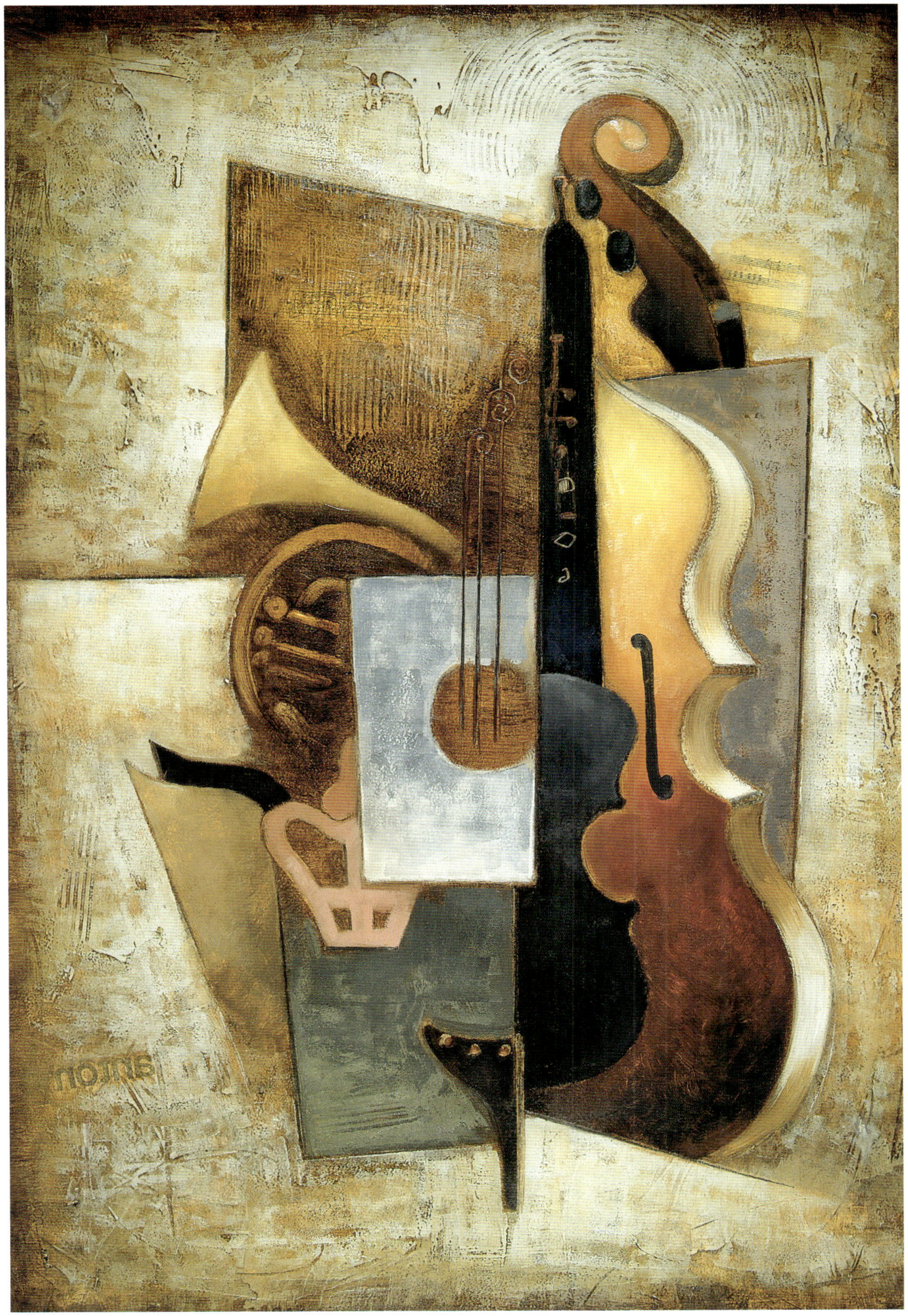

Orchestration
Orchestra Aura VI

Mixed Media on Canvas
30"x44"

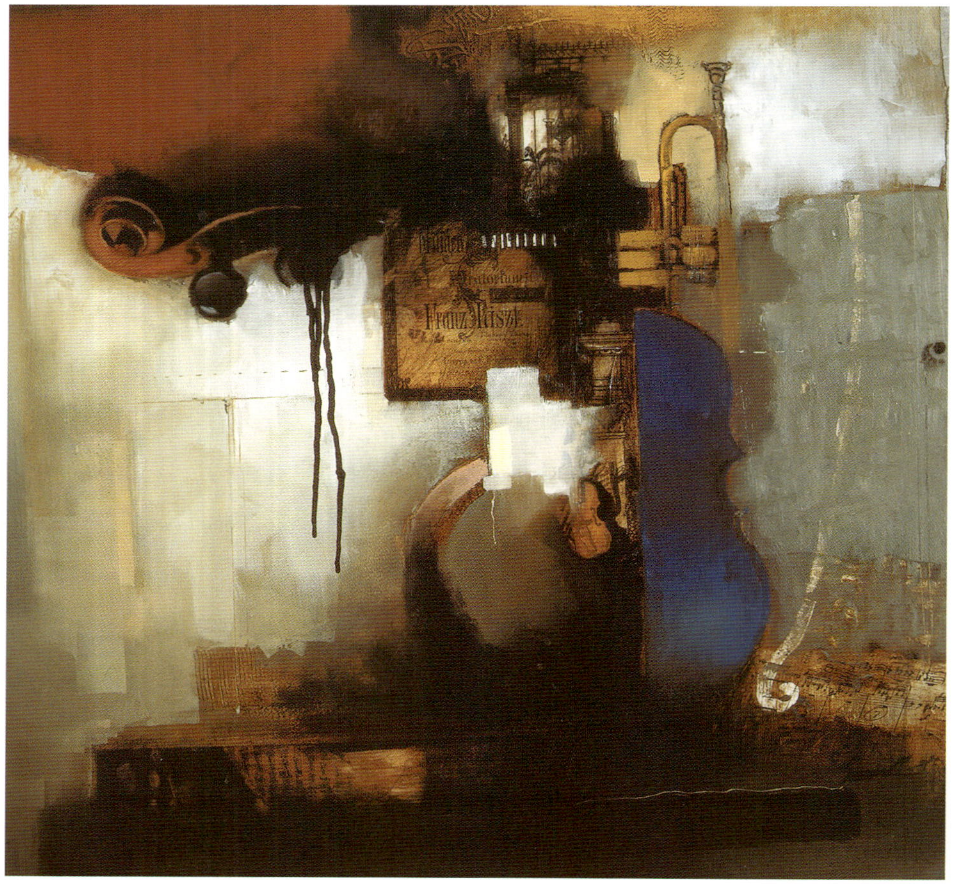

Why such a fascination with words?

I think the use of words and letters enriches art. Language and form are so different that I like to bring them together and make one like the other. Words become art and art takes on the role of language. Above all, words easily lose their meaning and become shopworn. I like to renew them through art. Art can re-energize their semantic purposes. I also like words because they are beautiful sculptures of sound and form.

Melodium
Metro Sonata I

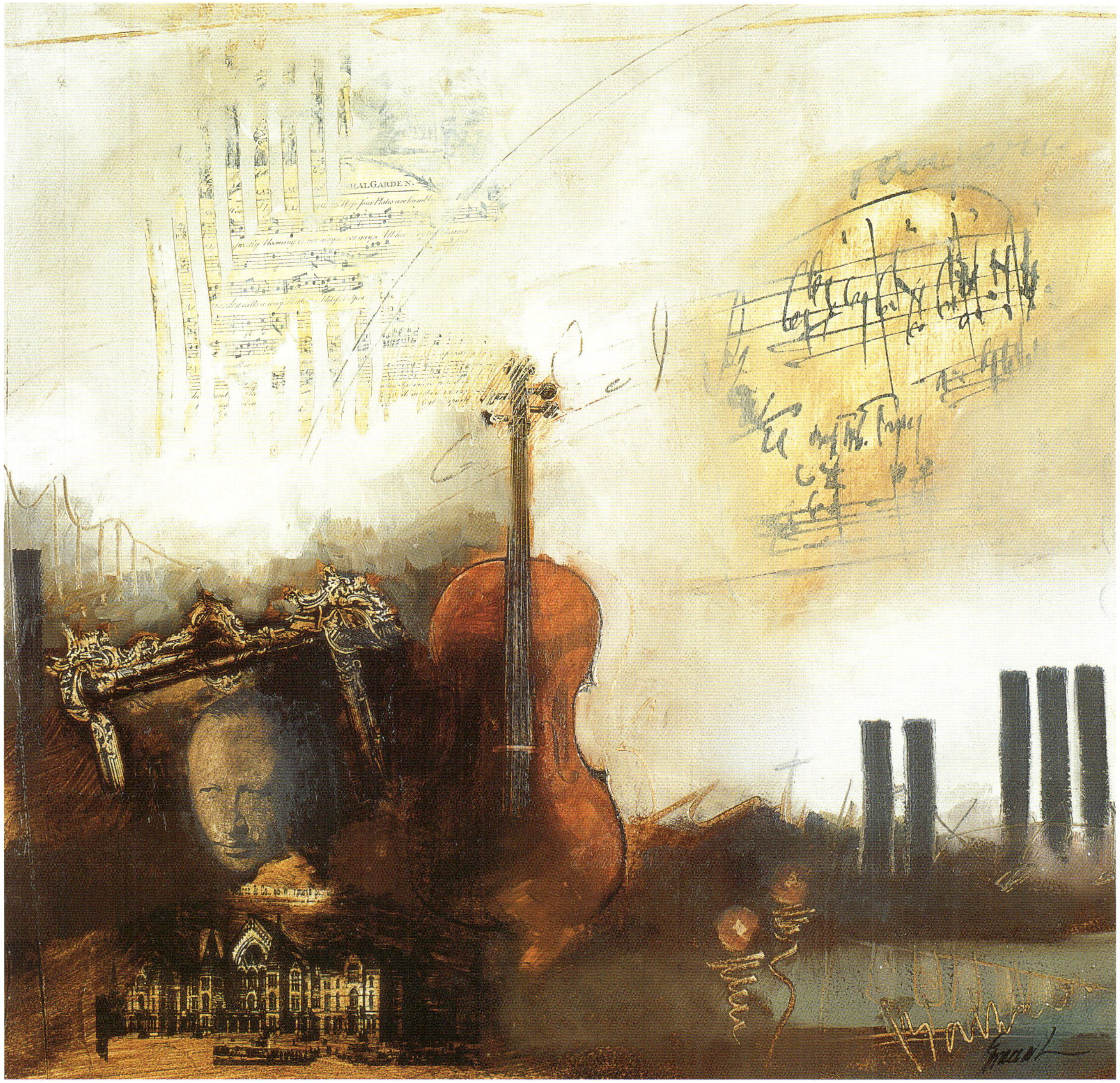

Melodium
Metro Sonata II

Mixed Media on Paper 20"x20"

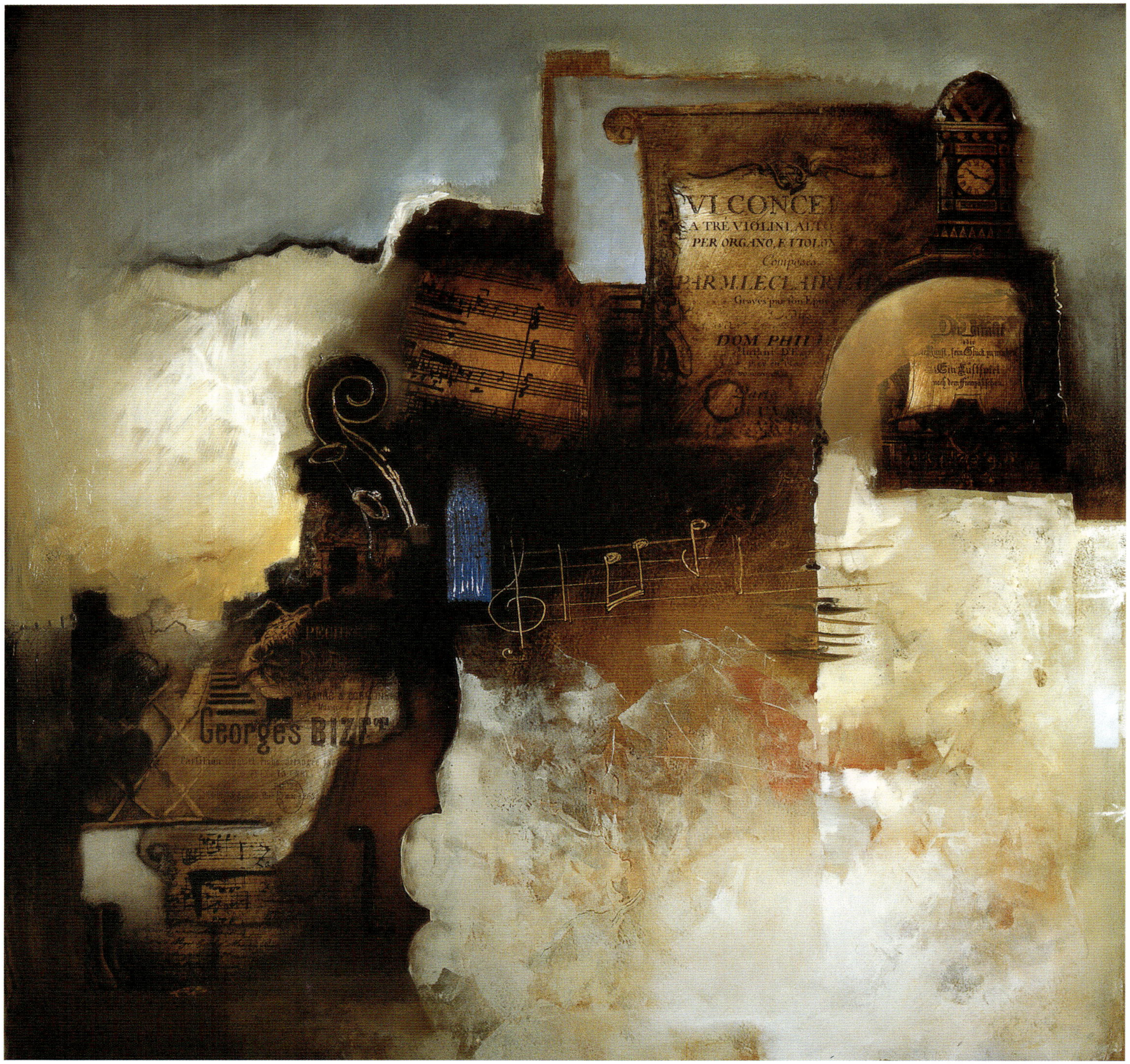

Melodium
Metro Sonata III

Mixed Media on Paper 30"x30"

"I want to go beyond what is visibly obvious and find the spirit that moves what we see."

Given that words and letters of the alphabet have also been a part of the western tradition of paintings since the early 1900s, do you see a merging of the western and eastern traditions in today's art?

It has taken the West many centuries to acknowledge the beauty of letters and of calligraphy. And the East is becoming more individuated in terms of its expressions.

I am perplexed by the plurality of your style.
You seem to traverse a wide range of ideas and visions.

I am interested in the history of man's aesthetics. I am not only concerned with expressing myself, but I also want to learn from the various languages of expression to further my own artistic pursuits.

This seems to be one major attribute of Postmodernism often referred to as appropriation.
Are you consciously guided by this principle?

Not consciously, but we are all part of our own age and we cannot escape its demands upon us. In one sense, we cannot help but appropriate. At the same time, it is impossible to exactly copy.

What do you seek in and through your art?

This is a tough question. I suppose I seek the simplicity of nature. The elemental powers that reduce multiple forms into a single sensation. I want to go beyond what is visibly obvious and find the spirit that moves what we see.

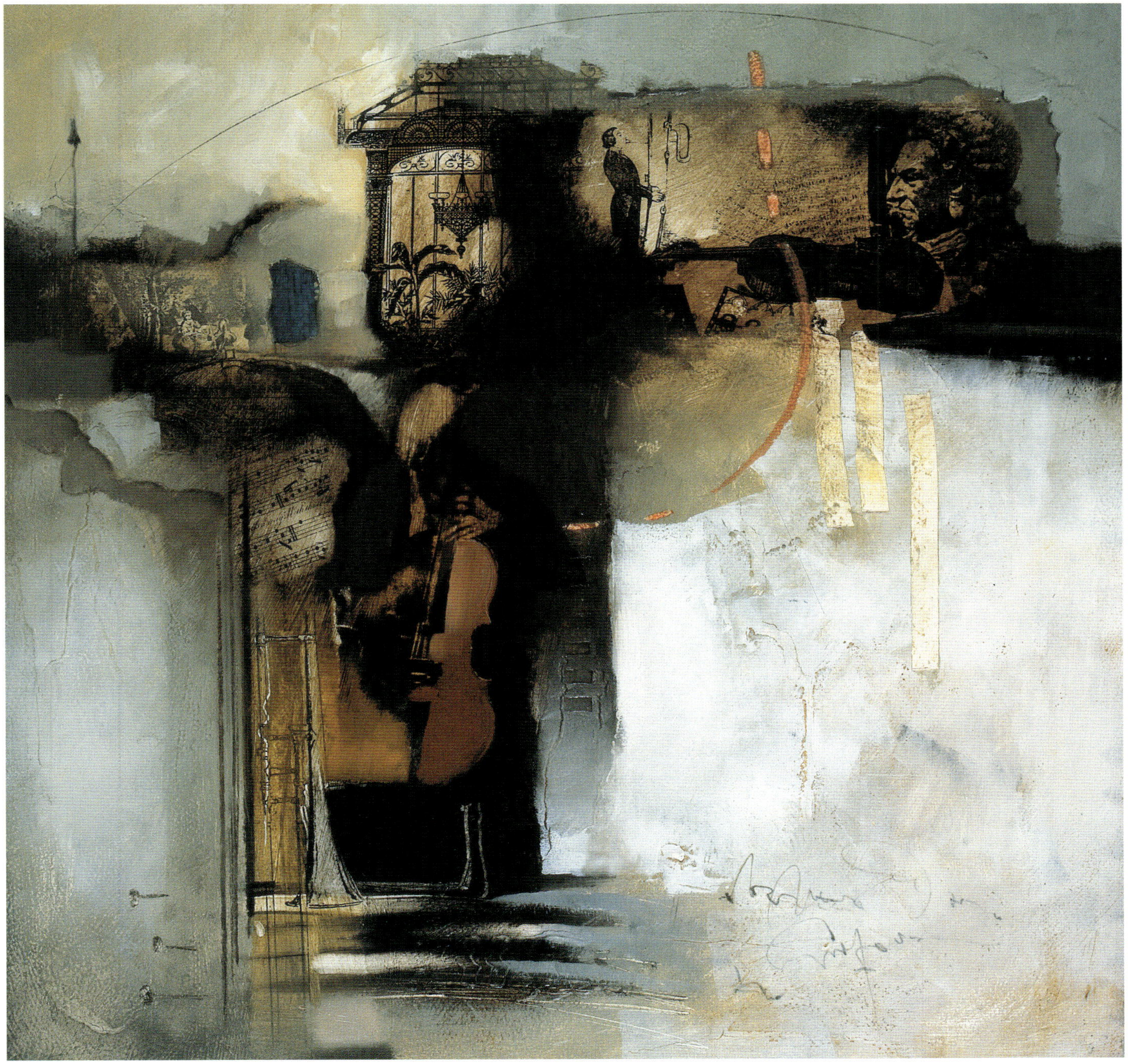

Melodium
Metro Sonata IV

Mixed Media on Paper 20"x20"

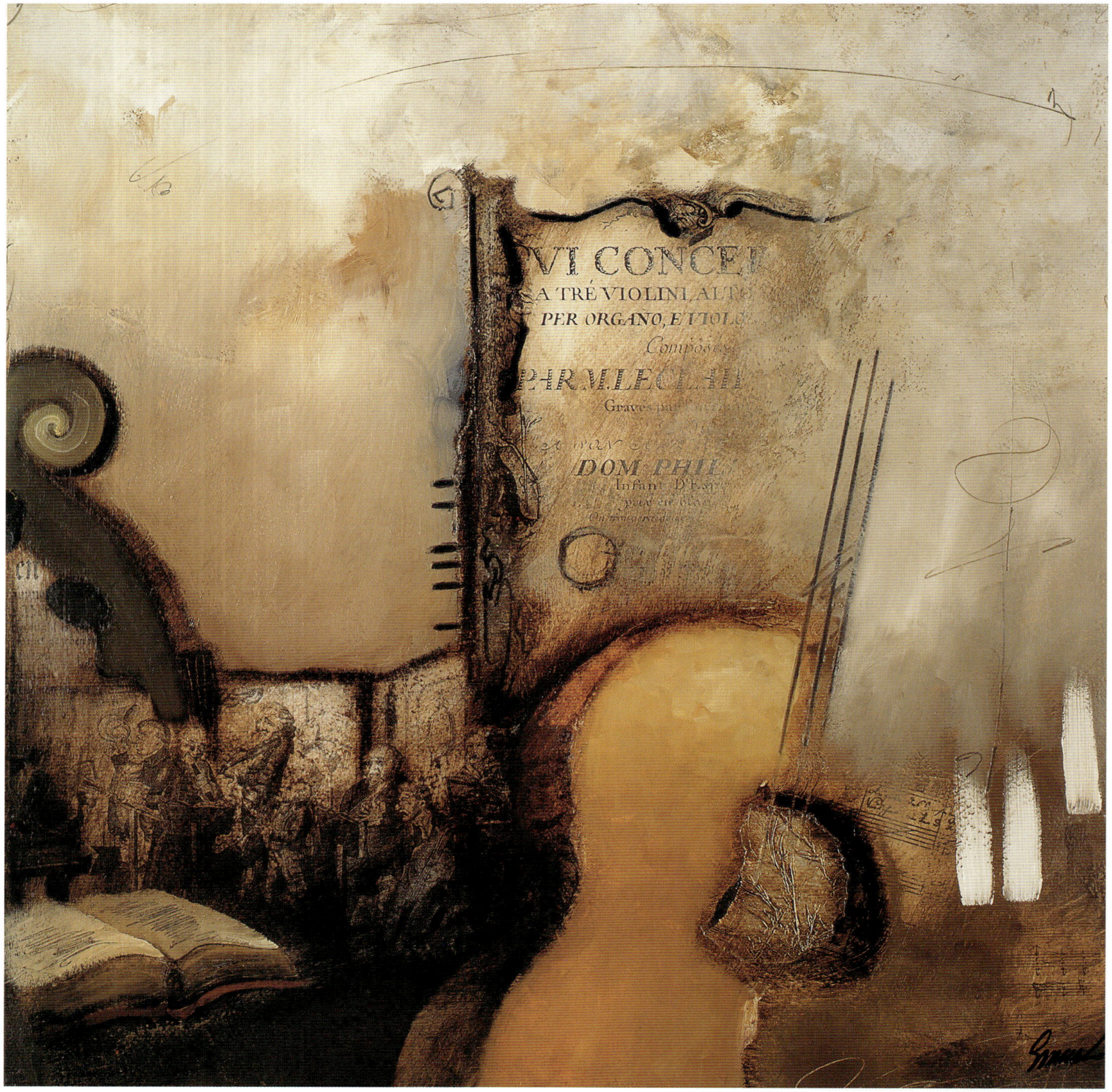

Melodium Incantata I

Mixed Media on Paper 20"x20"

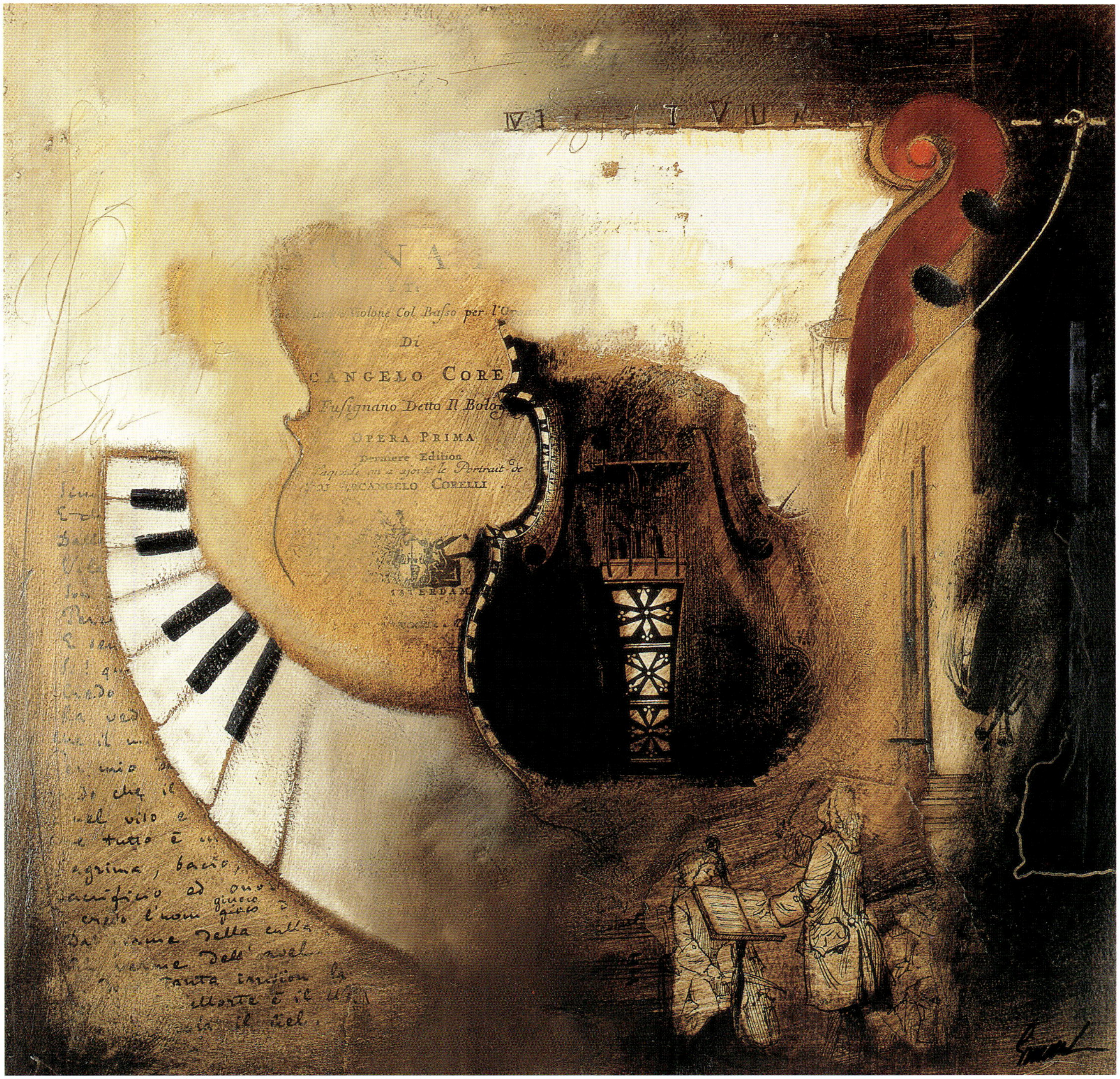

Melodium
Solano Winter I

Mixed Media on Paper
20"x20"

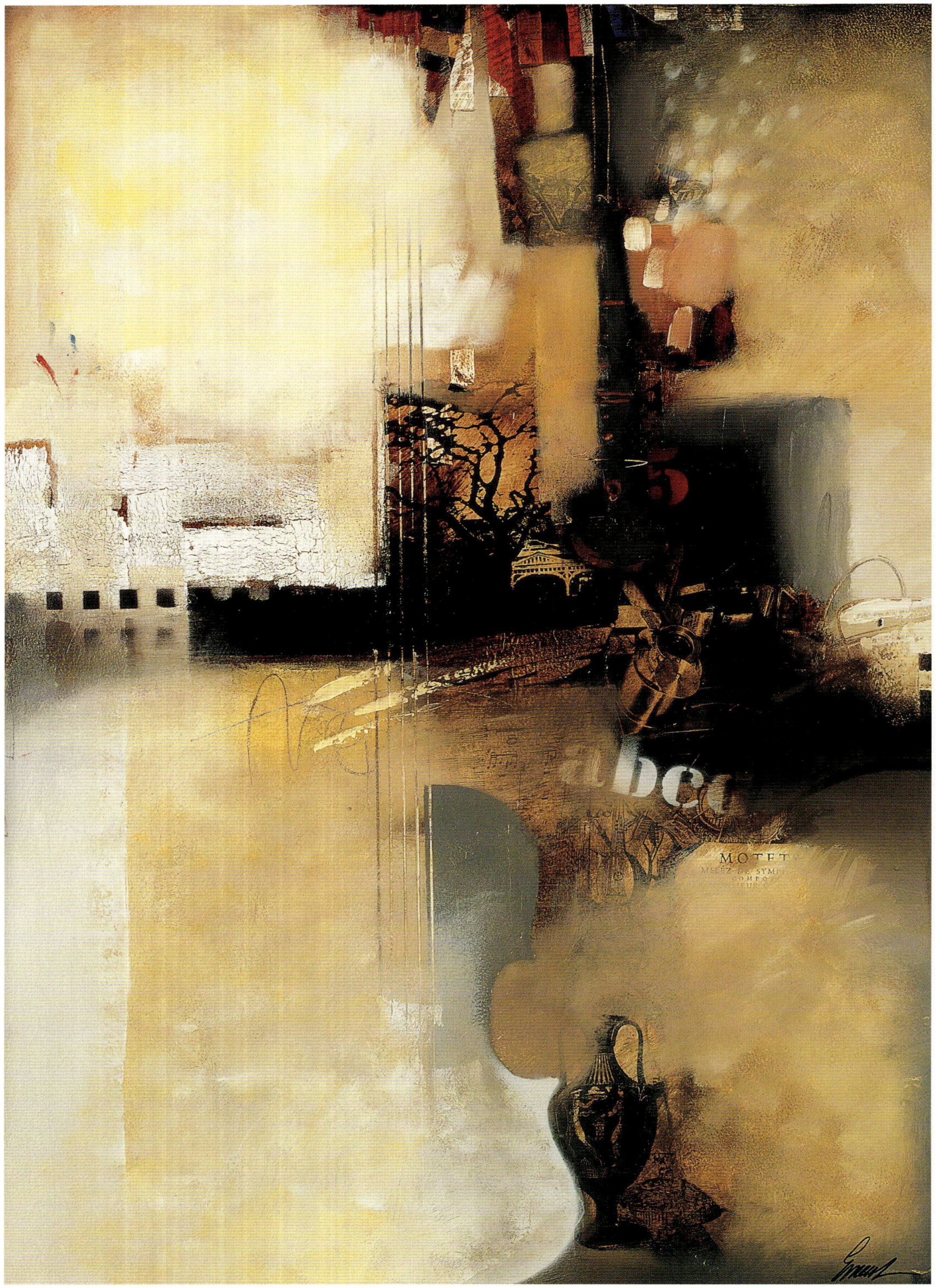

Melodium
Solano Summer I

Mixed Media on Canvas 40"x54"

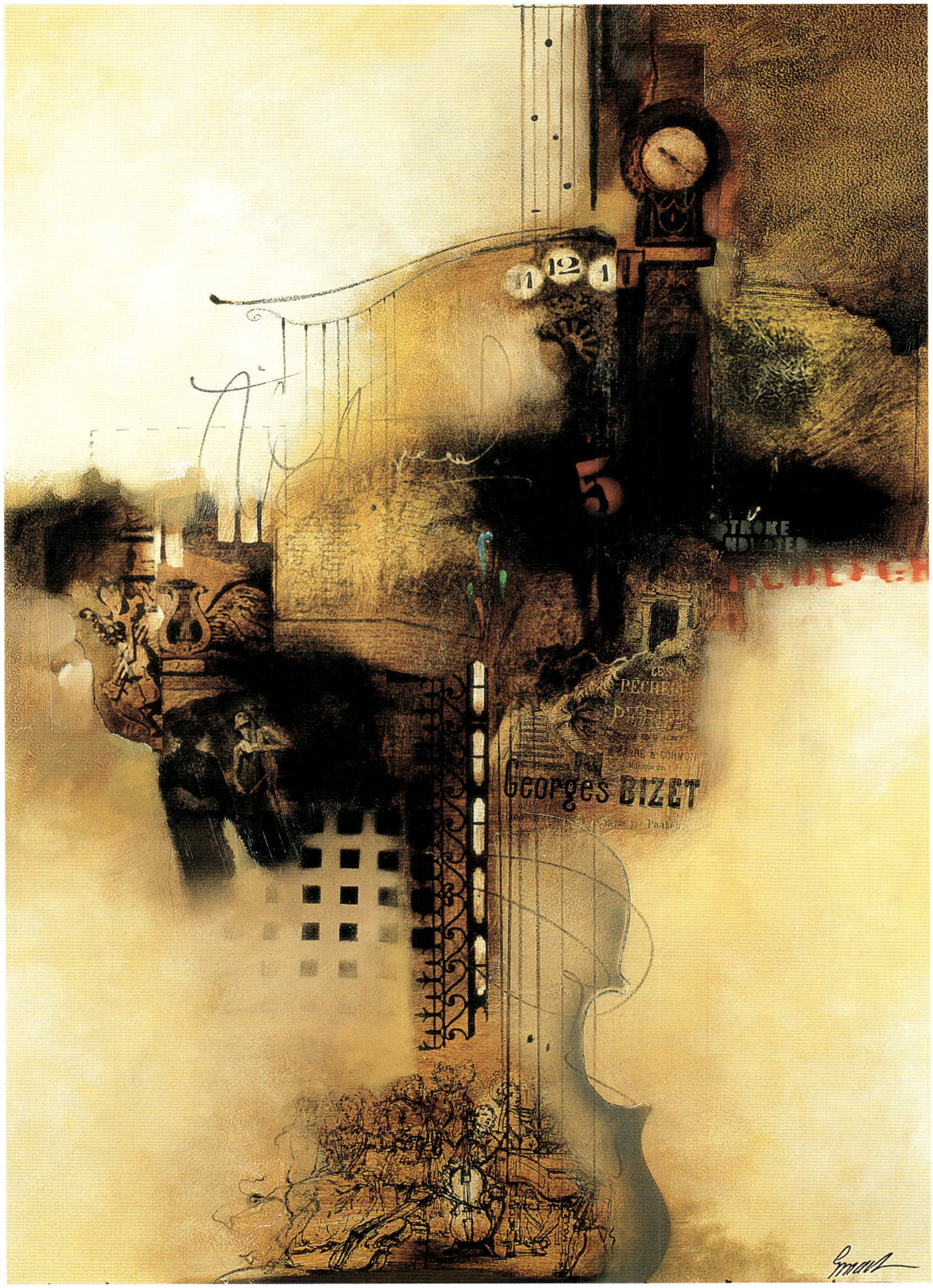

Melodium
Solano Summer II

Mixed Media on Canvas 40"x54"

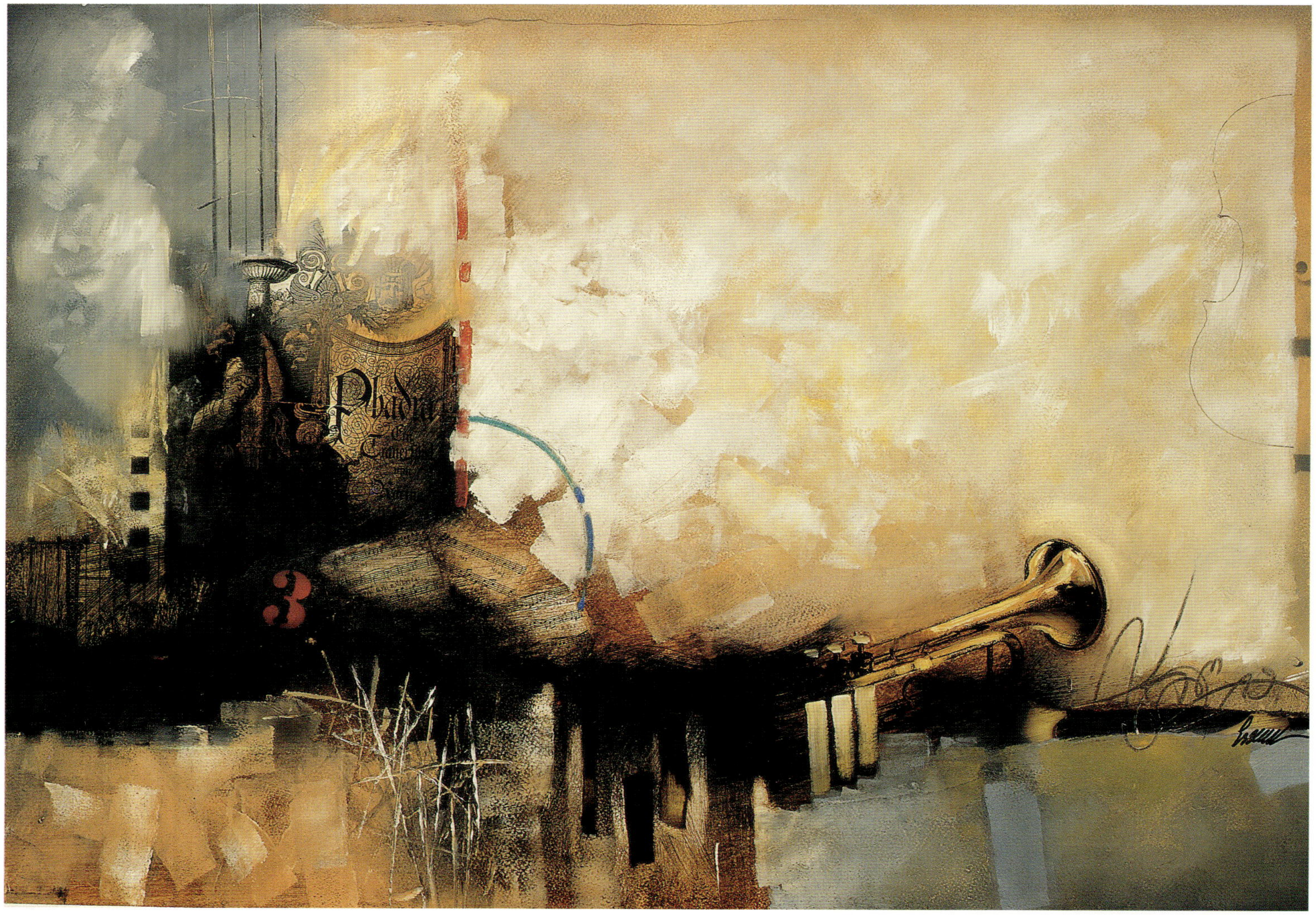

Melodium
Soft Etude I

Mixed Media on Canvas 54"x40"

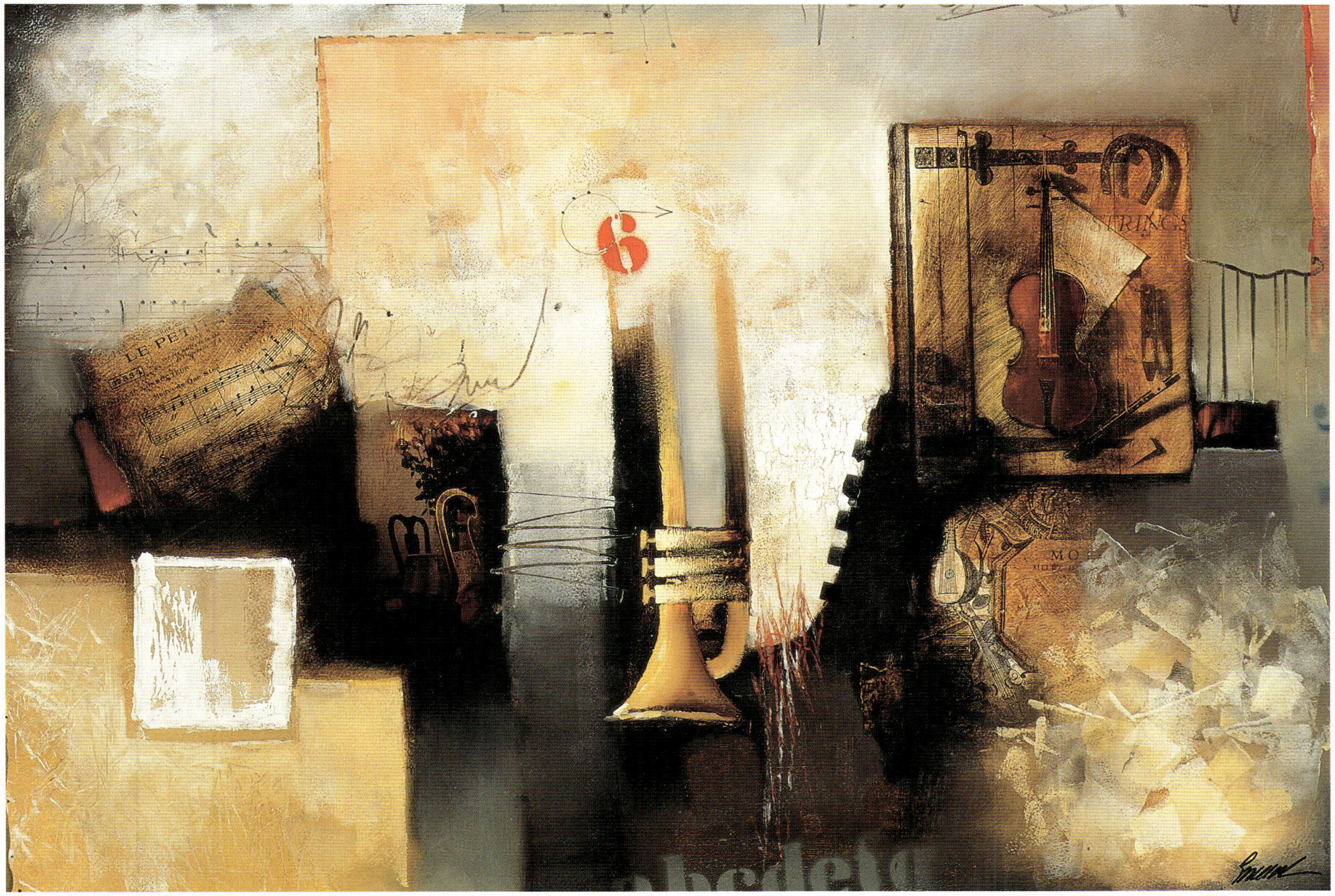

Melodium
Soft Etude II

Mixed Media on Canvas 54"x40"

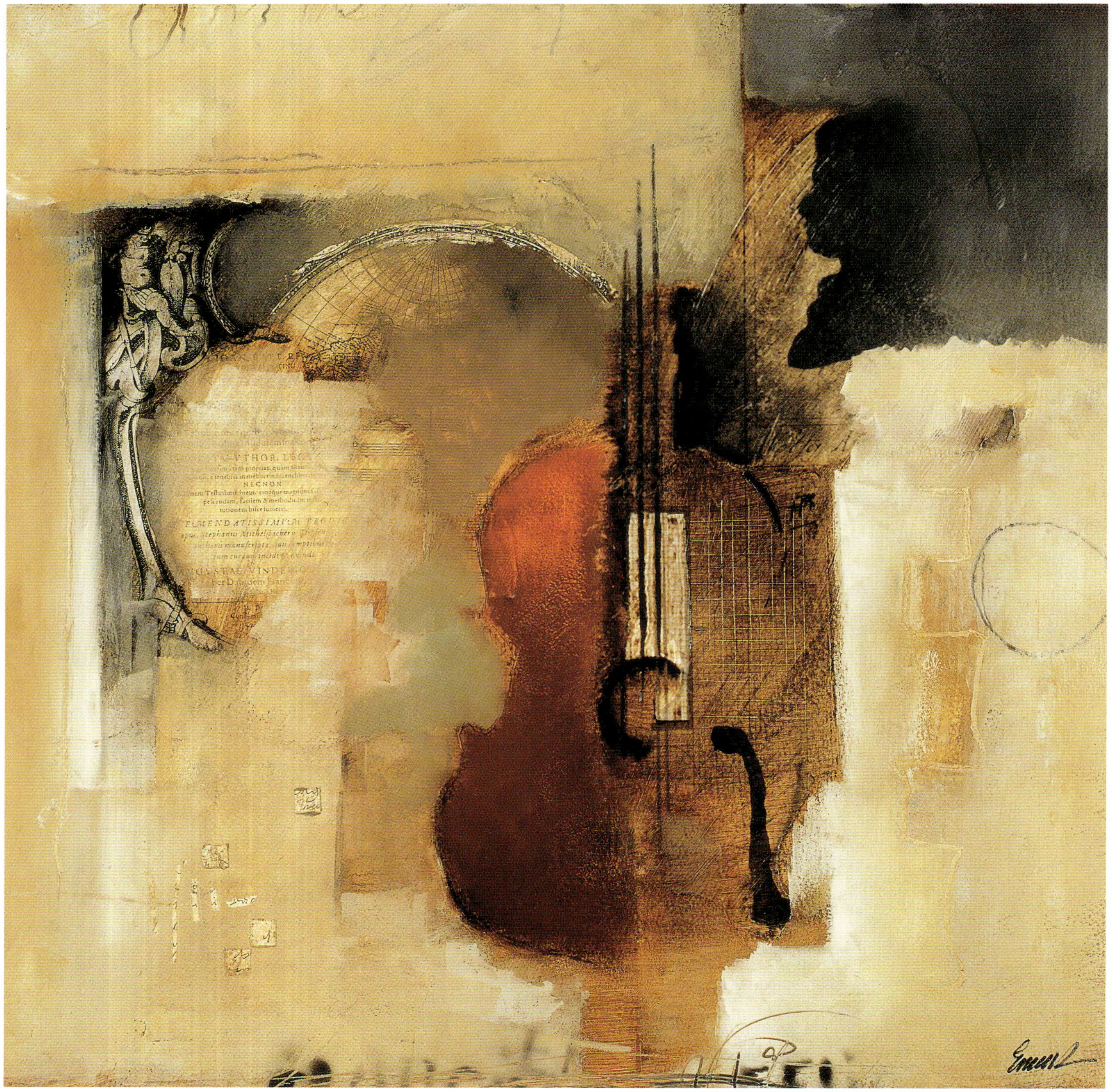

Melodium Principia Etude I

Mixed Media on Paper 20"x20"

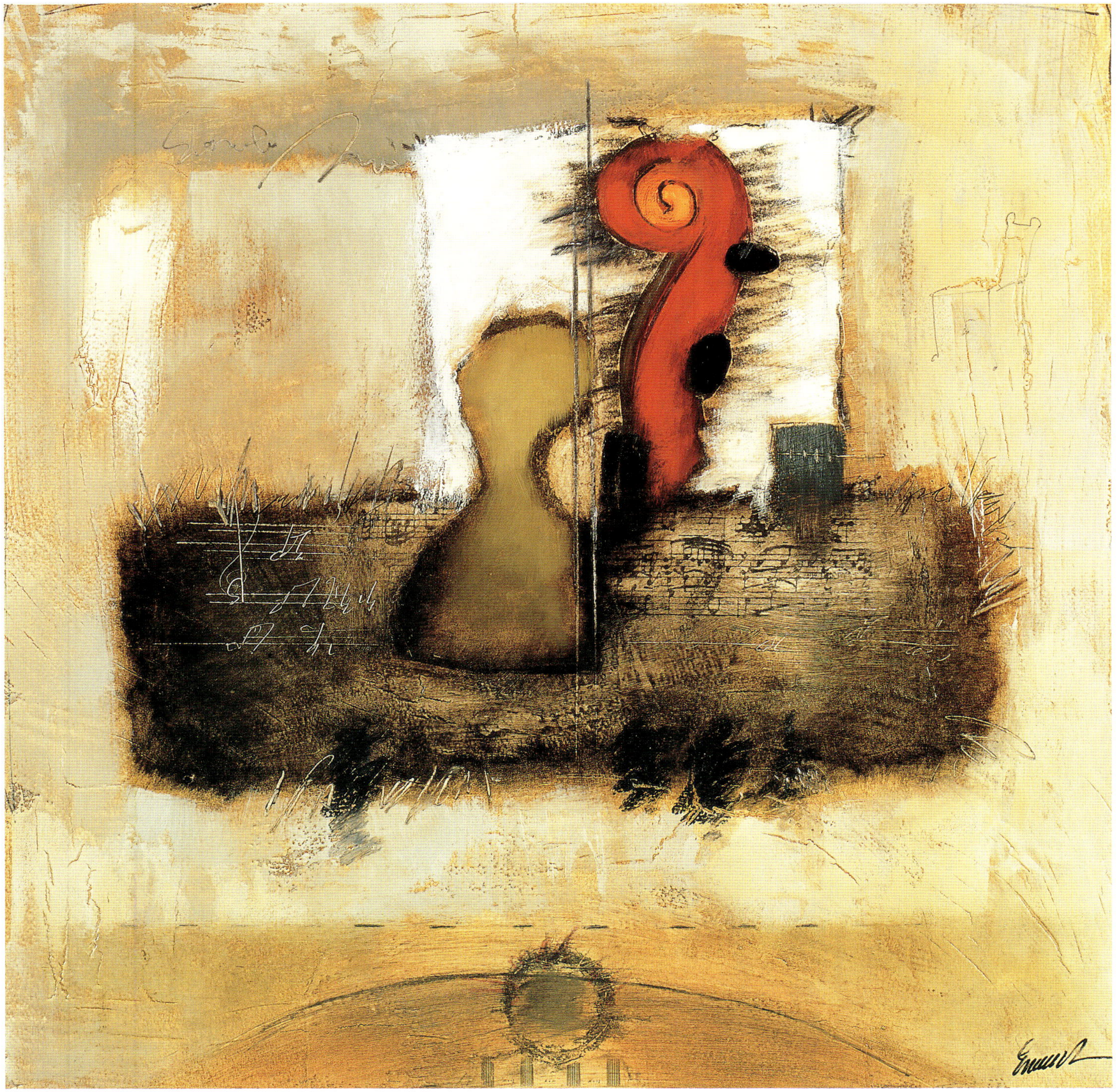

Melodium
Principia Etude II

Mixed Media on Paper 20"x20"

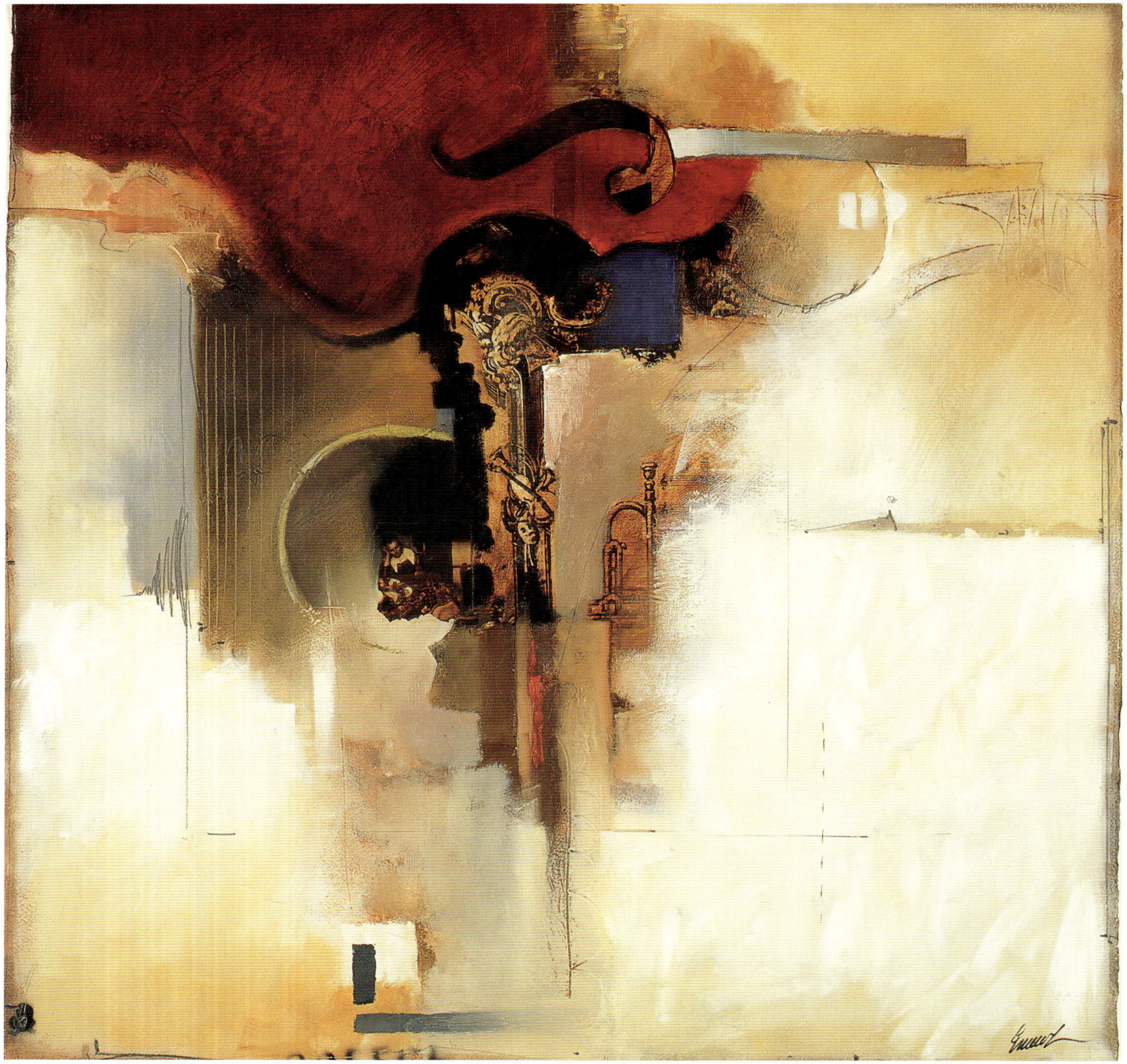

Melodium
Principia Etude III

Mixed Media on Paper 20"x20"

Essay

The Paintings

"The artist is the antennae of the race."

Ezra Pound

# of Emanuel

by Abbas Daneshvari, Ph.D.

"There are two kinds of artists—revolu
and plagiarists."

Paul Gauguin

Introduction

In the 1980s, Corinne Robbins in an exemplary book coined the art of the second half of the twentieth century as **The Pluralistic Era**. Her book showed that the many faces and styles of art from the seventies to the nineties reflect and mirror the multiplicities of visions that have permeated the mind and body of the western cultures. There is now a consensus that at the end of this long journey from modern to postmodern the genius of the artist is more a matter of pluralities of vision and style rather than the focused perception of Modernism.

tionaries

Emanuel is truly an artist of this milieu. It is therefore not easy to write of his art because of complexities that, though partly born of the inexplicabilities of his personality, are nevertheless to a great extent a condition of the late twentieth century zeitgeist. For the western world, at the end of one millennium and on the threshold of another, is absorbing as much from the outside as it is itself absorbed into worlds that it once considered alien. The cultural and artistic assimilations that have produced synthetic Postmodernism speak on multifarious levels and address the many issues that have preoccupied the making and understanding of art in the last one hundred and fifty years. These issues, such as originality in art, subjective values versus objective truths and language versus abstraction, have permeated the form and spirit of art in the last quarter of the twentieth century.

They have led, philosophically and artistically, to conflations of diametrically opposed principles. Thinking and intuition, high and low art, art and anti-art meet to find a new vision. In some ways, because of these conflations, art at the end of the twentieth century reads like an anthology of aesthetic theory and a sampling of modernist aesthetics. Our complex age exacerbates the problems of understanding art in terms of neat and packaged ideas. Gauguin's world of revolutionaries and plagiarists no longer applies in the convoluted context of Postmodernism where mimesis (copying) is one method of communicating and expressing. It is interesting that Emanuel, especially as an artist born abroad, does not work within the narrow confines of eastern Romanticism or western Modernism. Clearly, he has not been immune to the vicissitudes of Postmodernism which are powerfully his western zeitgeist. His art, as discussed below, is indeed an aspect of what has been called multi-culturalism and the New Internationalism, thus making him an authentic and a relevant artist in his age.

When Ezra Pound said that "the artist is the antennae of the race," he was also addressing obliquely the question of authenticity of art and the genius of the artist. We cannot deny that authenticity of style and its relation to its social context will ultimately judge the art-form. Great art always mirrors its setting while others found to be irrelevant are buried in the dust piles of history. The fact that history acknowledges only those who are relevant and those who reveal the prevailing attitudes of their time is a truism because what stands is that which reflects the spirit of its time. Moreover, the many conflicting and antipodal aesthetic choices, given time, reveal that the changes in taste are really the

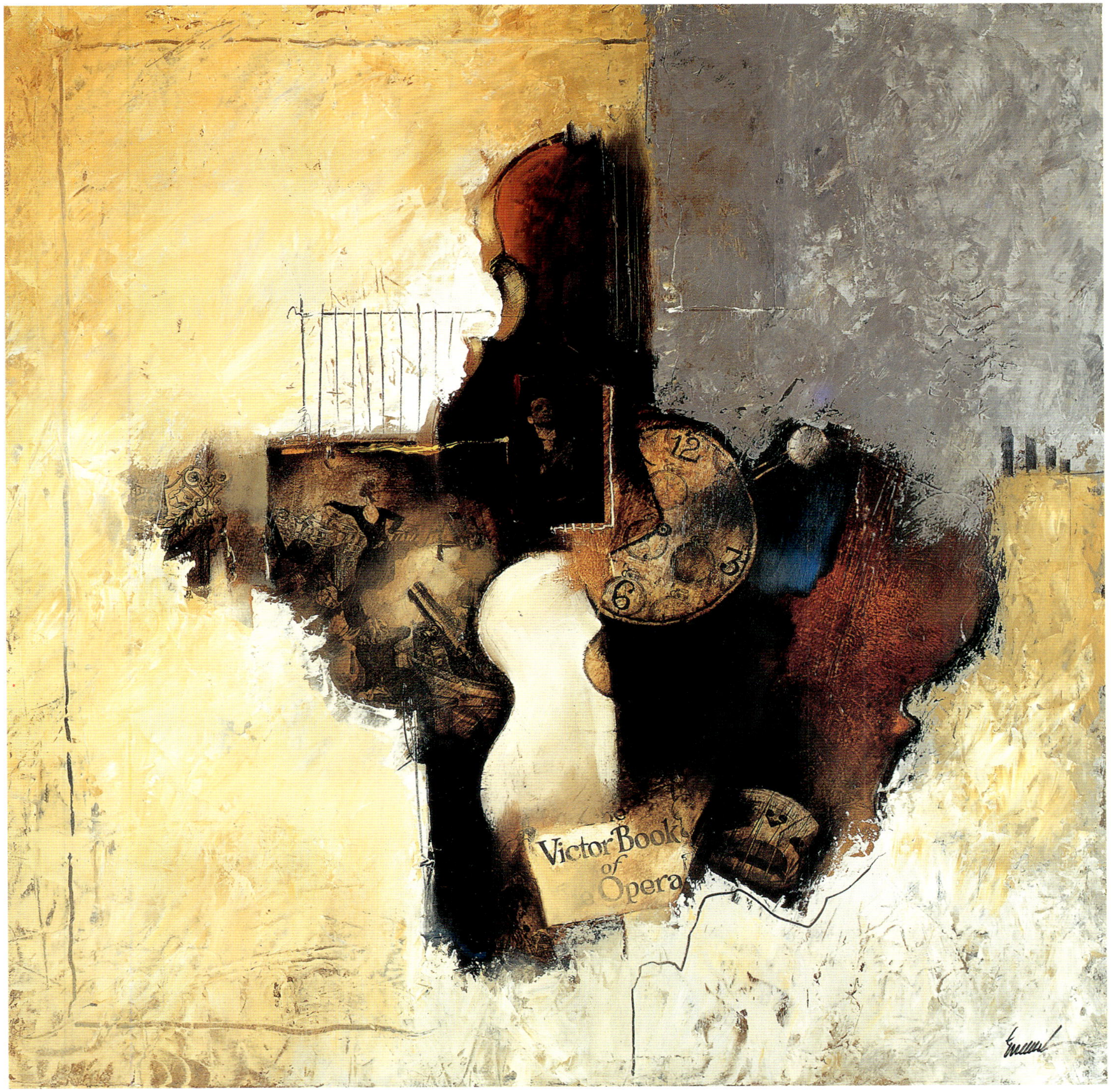

Melodium
Principia Etude IV

Mixed Media on Paper 20"x20"

changes in conditions of life. Historically speaking there is no absolute and no great art, only an act of referencing and indexing one's own time in depth and with enough breadth to allow the art to survive and thus represent its period. This is one reason why Emanuel's art is captivating, for it represents through its multifarious styles some of the tenets and dogmas of late twentieth century art and Postmodernism. In addition, while in certain regards a modernist, there is an inextricable and fascinating dimension of his art which calls into question the judicious standards of Modernism. These questions and doubts evoked by his art enable him as a commentator on the life and beliefs of the late twentieth century. On a subconscious level, he makes us focus on the excesses and pitfalls of our decadent materialism, while a few of his romantic paintings address kitsch and the end of art.

Therefore, one of my core concerns has been to illuminate his stylistic relationships with the many sources that have engendered them, be they western or eastern, modern or pre-modern. I will investigate the manner in which the shifting geographies of his life cycles have inevitably contributed to the richness of his varied stylistic expressions and add to the depth of his emotional perspectives. I hope to show that Emanuel's art benefits from a polarity that also complicates it. It traverses from Modernism and Abstraction to Romanticism and Idealism. **"Orchestration,"** for example, stands in sharp contrast to **"Hallycon,"** and likewise the collage techniques of **"Passages"** are a far cry from the transcendent abstractions of **"Melodium, Metro Sonata."** The former is cerebral while the latter is poetic, fluid and even romantic in a deeply subjective and solipsistic way.

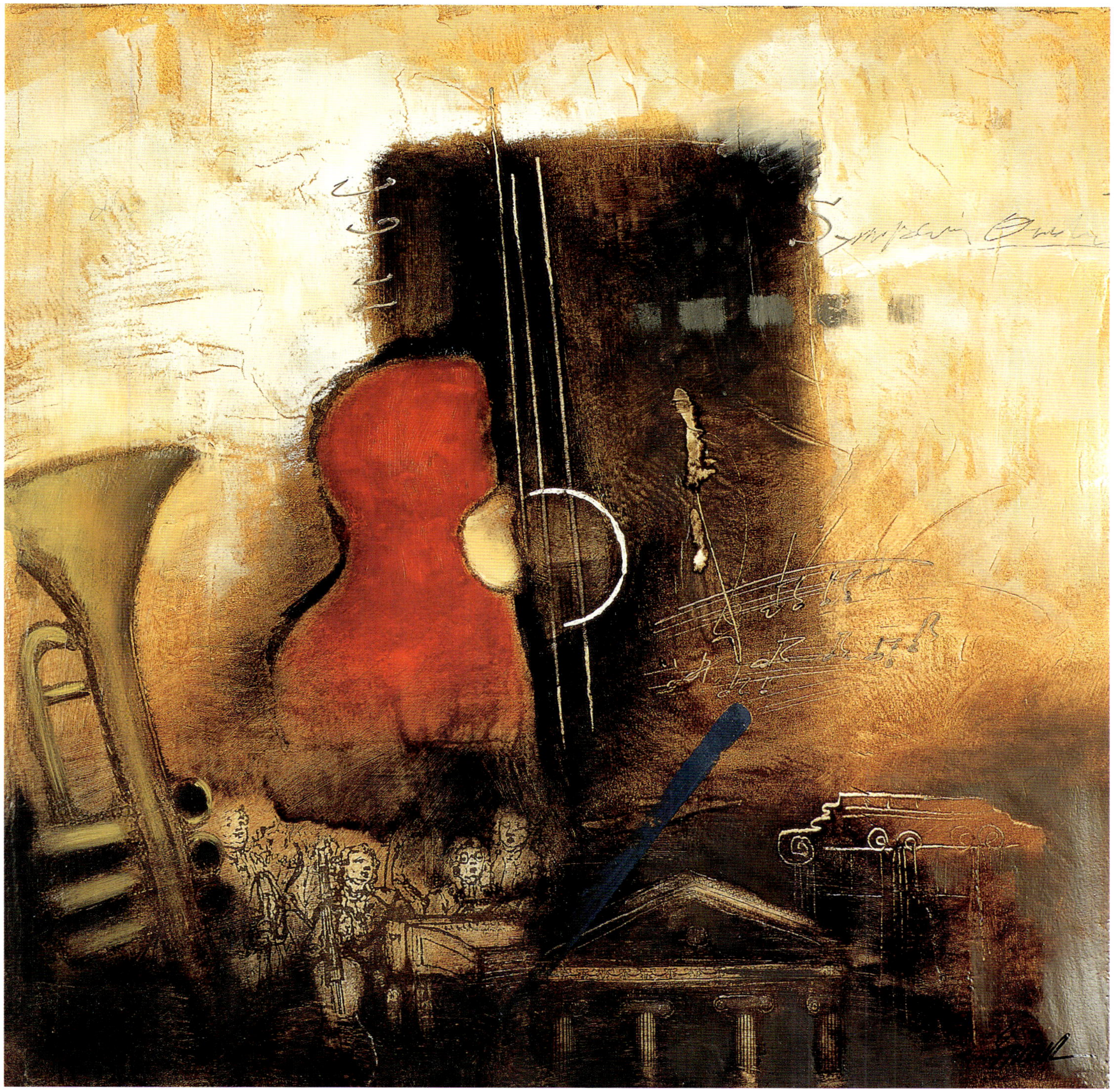

Melodium
Principia Etude V

Mixed Media on Paper 20"x20"

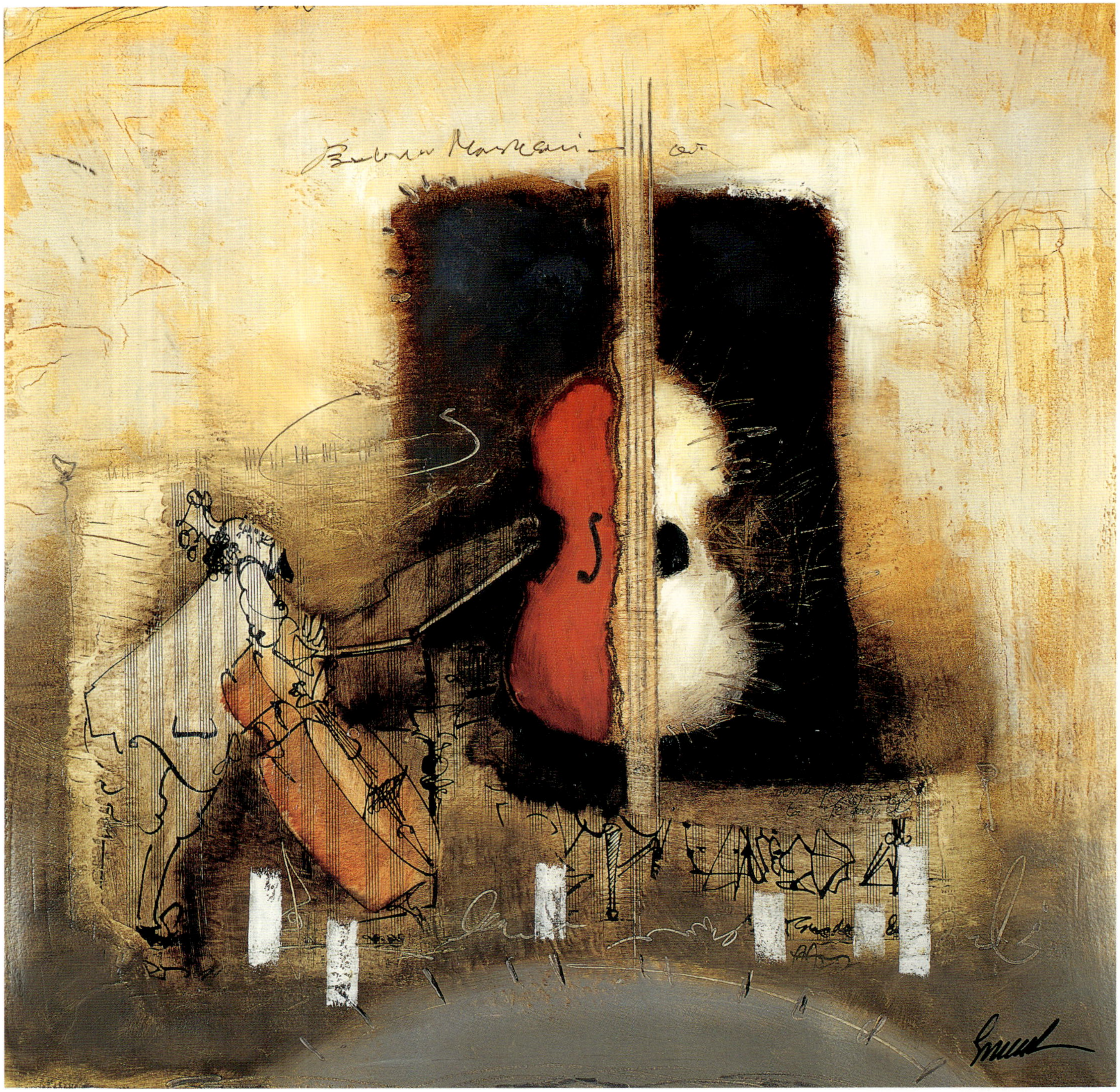

Melodium Profundis I

Mixed Media on Paper 20"x20"

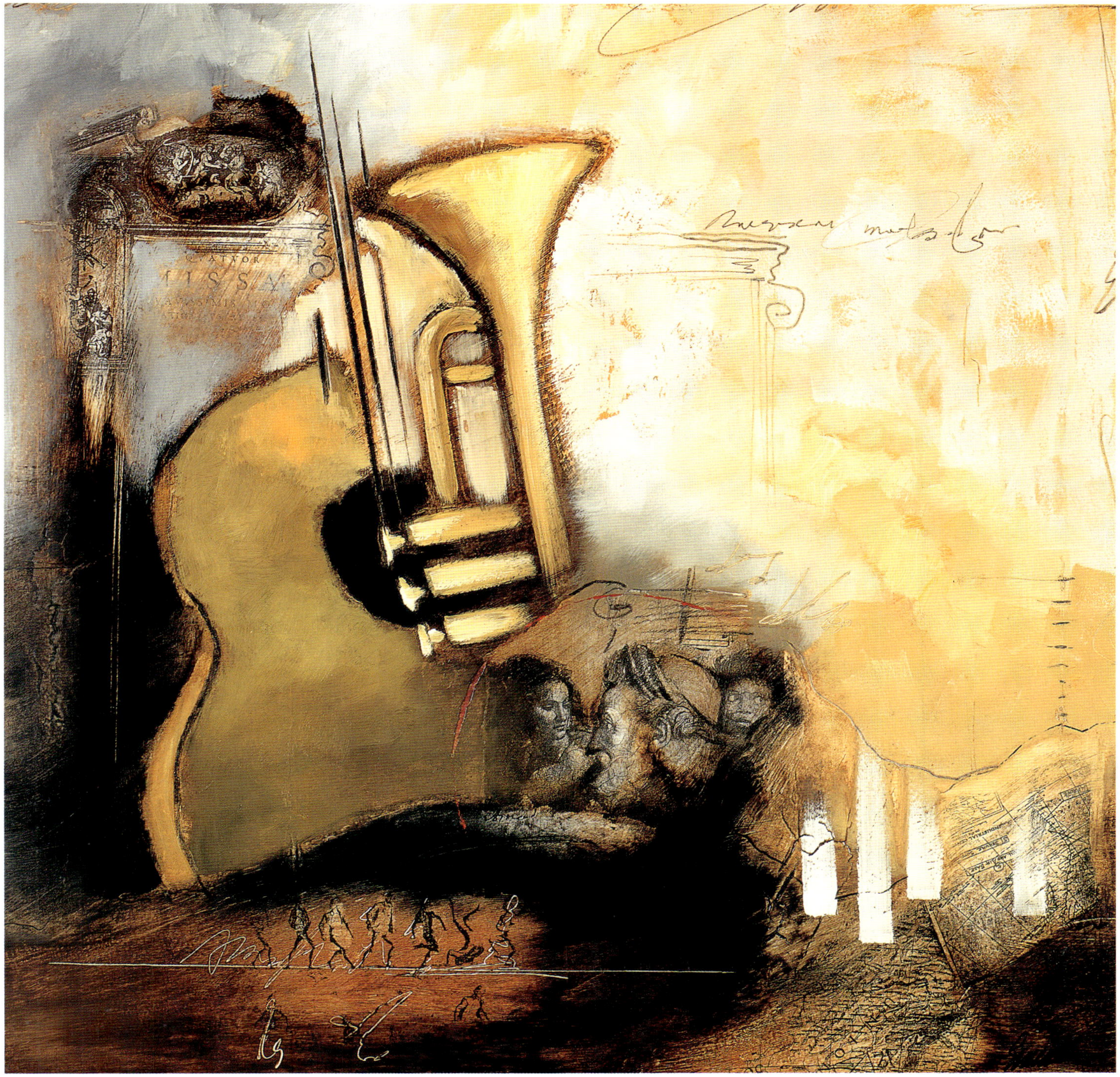

Melodium Profundis II

Mixed Media on Paper 20"x20"

"The past has a tyrannic which is difficult to escape... ...The worst is that there is always something of the past within us."

Piet Mondrian

From Language To Freedom: The Road To Abstraction

Language is memory. It carries the past into the present and, though we are reluctant to admit, also the past into the future. For the Austrian Philosopher Ludwig Wittgenstein, language was a kind of prison that killed individuality and unique subjectivity. Language is a consensual, and in the arts a mimetic form, which reproduces and presents itself in many guises. It suffers from the rigidity of its own logos and

influence

dialectical operation. Abstraction on the other hand is presentation. It denies the past and attempts to reach primal revelations. For many, abstraction was and is the pathway to freedom, to an expression independent of memory and past interference. Memory is abstraction's greatest enemy, for it eschews the primal and abhors the absence of consensual signification.

There is no doubt that one of the purposes of art is to strive for absolute freedom and present a desire to move beyond the quotidian and the superficial, perhaps wishing to recognize a truth beneath the world of appearances. This drive for freedom found its strongest expression in the modern age, propelled by individuation and the desire to explore the mysterious subconscious. The gateway to these artistic and ontological mutations was abstraction and the defiance of the conventional languages of expression and communication. In the history of modern art varying degrees of abstraction correlate to varying degrees of liberation from the objective world. The process signals the degrees by which the world of reality and language is transformed into sensations. From the abstract forms radiate energies from a world free of historically bound interpretations and historical demands.

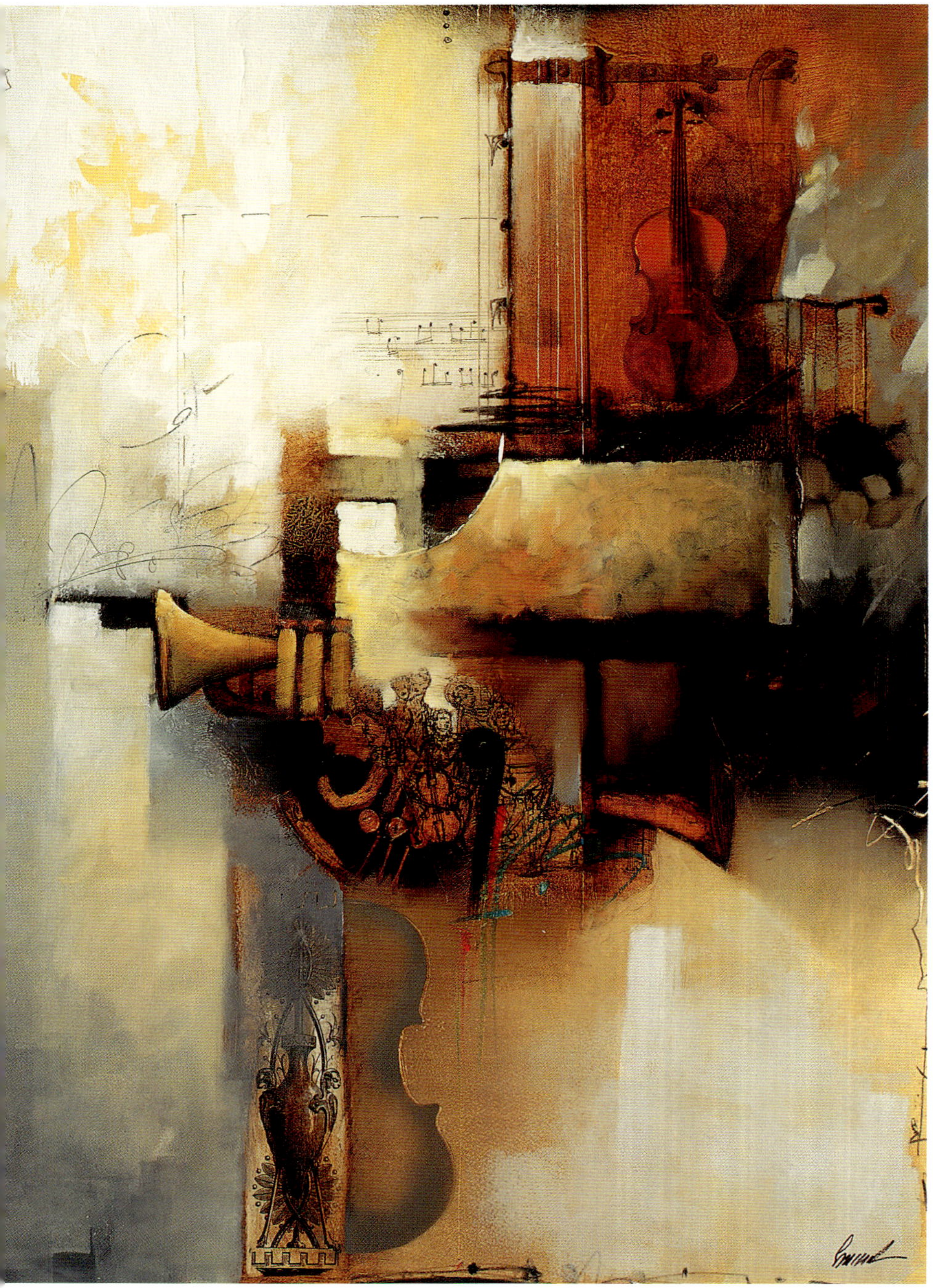

For Emanuel, the pathways towards abstraction began with archetypal imagery and evolved into a full and complete transcendence beyond the image. His "**Orchestration**"[59-79] series, for example, is a quest for the archetypal musical context. Each and every one of the paintings in this series is a variation on the universal theme of instrumentation. Densely packed instruments create an overwhelming sense of their allegorical presence. This issue is further intensified by Emanuel's fondness to paint **en serie**, which as a method radiates multiple visions of being. In these paintings, fragments of instruments are piled high and evoke a strong gravitational wave, binding the objects tightly together. The forms, while distinct, also collapse onto a center whose density is high and weighty. The instruments wrap themselves in a dance alluding to underlying harmonies that breathe life into them. The distortions of the images, the twisting and turning of the forms, create the illusion of a space that rational scrutiny denies. The simplicity of forms and the complexity of design are reminders of the earlier works of Cubists, whose compositions signaled the rise of a new order of vision and thinking.

The "**Orchestration**" landscapes, with their tonal variations, signal the beginning of the end of the object in Emanuel's paintings. They represent a step or even a movement toward a universe of pure sensations, toward viewing art as a process rather than as an objective end product. They promote feeling and sensations over objectified sight, and prefer the irrational arrangements that connote unbounded space defying time and material tangibility. These works will lead us to the dark veils of his abstractions and the mysteries of the world rather than the reality of objects. In time, Emanuel's artistic temperament rejects the narrow and limited scope of language and consciousness and opts for such works as seen in **"Precis I."**[21] These abstractions become the very battlefield of silence and sound. But the sounds no longer tell a story that is conventionally communicable.

"Orchestration" owes a great deal to Modernism. Its arrangements are not subordinated to the linear-chronological and the recessional. Forms come together as notes of music and the complexities of the works make the reading of the images diachronic, rather than the customary synchronic readings possible in paintings. In addition, the shapes of the canvases when seen as a group, because of their many variations, evoke a musical dance which enhances the diachronic signification.

The **"Concerto"**[32-48] series, all at 20x20 inches, represents a slightly different vision of Emanuel's road to abstraction. The paintings of this series are suspended between the object and its absences. Forms or objects are transformed by their settings. The instruments are provided with contexts that transubstantiate them. Where in **"Orchestration"** the densely packed forms create a sense of two-dimensionality and of horror vacuii, in **"Concerto"** the space opens into infinity. Here the baroque amplitude of the **"Orchestration"** series gives way to a more austere arrangement that derives its emotional power from its setting. The gothic light of these settings, absent in **"Orchestration,"** imparts a sense of religious and devotional significance. **"Concerto VI"**[34] is simple

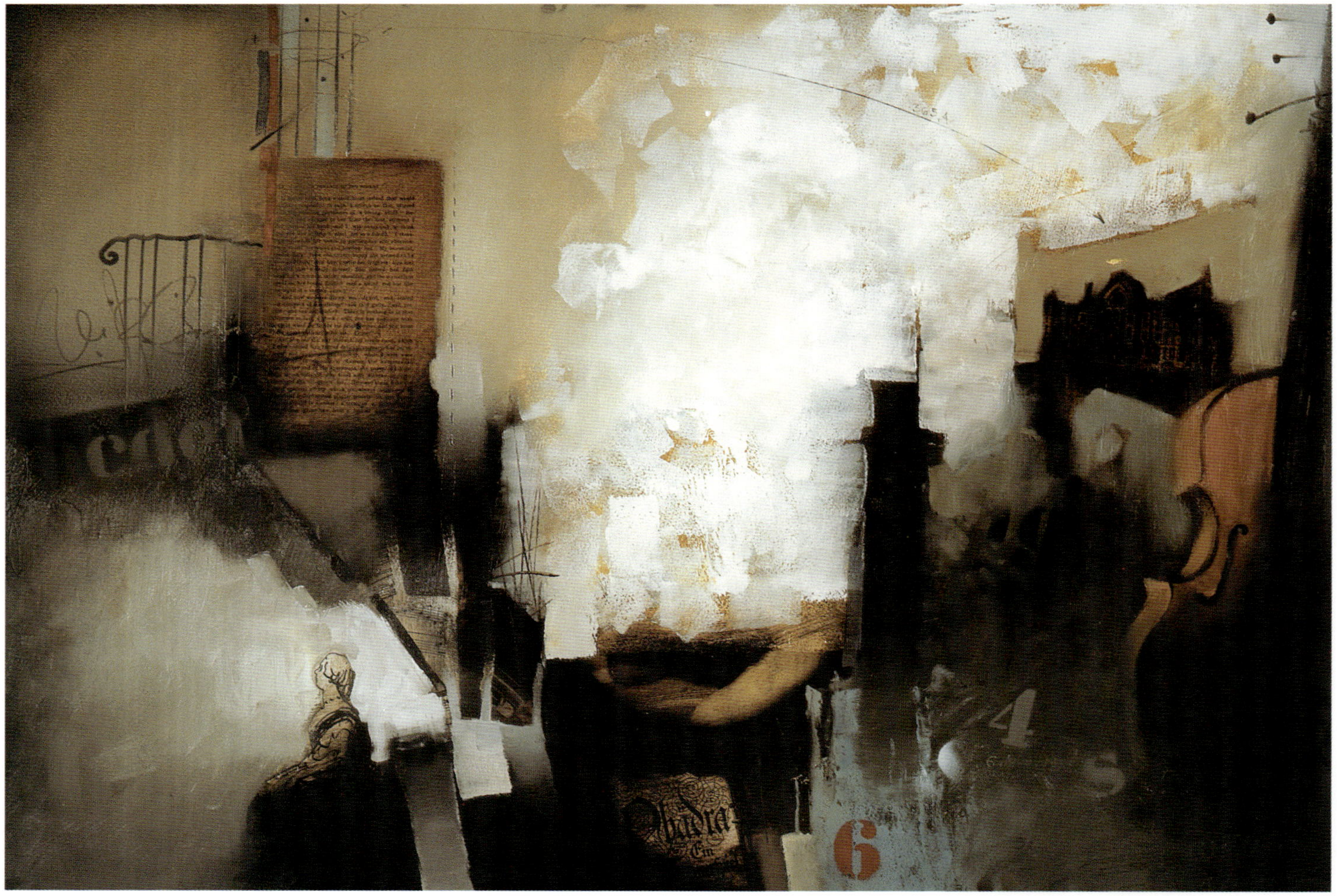

Investigation Poetica III

Mixed Media on Canvas 36"x24"

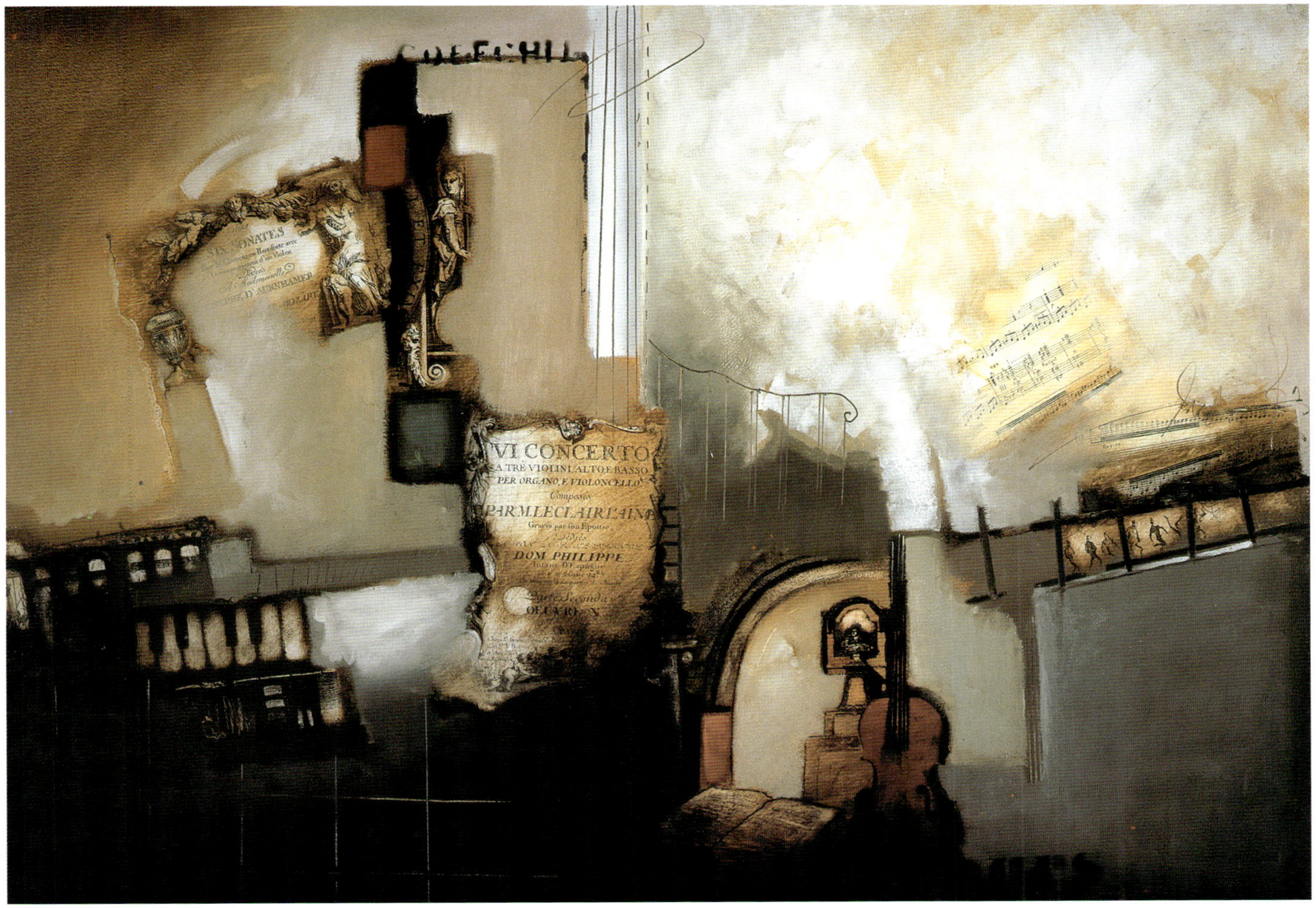

Investigation Poetica IV

Mixed Media on Canvas 34"x24"

and yet potent in terms of its implications; it offers a coherent picture of passion, ecstasies and piety. The image exists in simply constructed terms and yet its emotional powers are immense. There are mannerist aspects in these works that elevate themselves into worlds of conflict and anxiety. Here the flesh has been replaced by some ephemeral presence whose powers lie in the imagined domains rather than in the world of experience and reality. The illusion of infinity is at work in each of the **"Concerto"** paintings. These paintings speak with a solemn voice about some mysterious divinity that is music.

For every artist the process of change and realization is fraught with difficulties that are best exemplified in their transitional works. **"Ledger Line"**[21-31] and **"Appellation"**[18-19] are further forays toward abstraction and represent

"Seek those that constitute the the **lion** and the **Harlot** and the

the edge of Emanuel's transcendentalist paintings. **"Ledger Line"** is graphic and benefits from an austerity and simplicity that evokes a sense of primordial genesis for its musical instruments. We are placed at the dawn of their creation where shadowy figures rise from the void. The forms, appearing in bits and parts, are lyrical and appealing to the sensorium. The images are bathed in a shimmering light in which the energies of their colors are released. The **"Ledger Line"** paintings, more than any other of Emanuel's series, approach what the Orphists such as Robert Delaunay and Frantiscek Kupka sought in their paintings: sound.

The morphically abbreviated musical images of **"Ledger Line"** have inordinate powers to evoke musical sensations. For Emanuel, the choice of musical imagery is not accidental. The images give rise to a semiological picture as the musical signs necessarily plant the idea of musical sound. The harmonies are, however, communicated with mannerist-like dances of forms that extend and expand into every direction and dimension. These attributes make the **"Ledger Line"** series in some ways iconic.

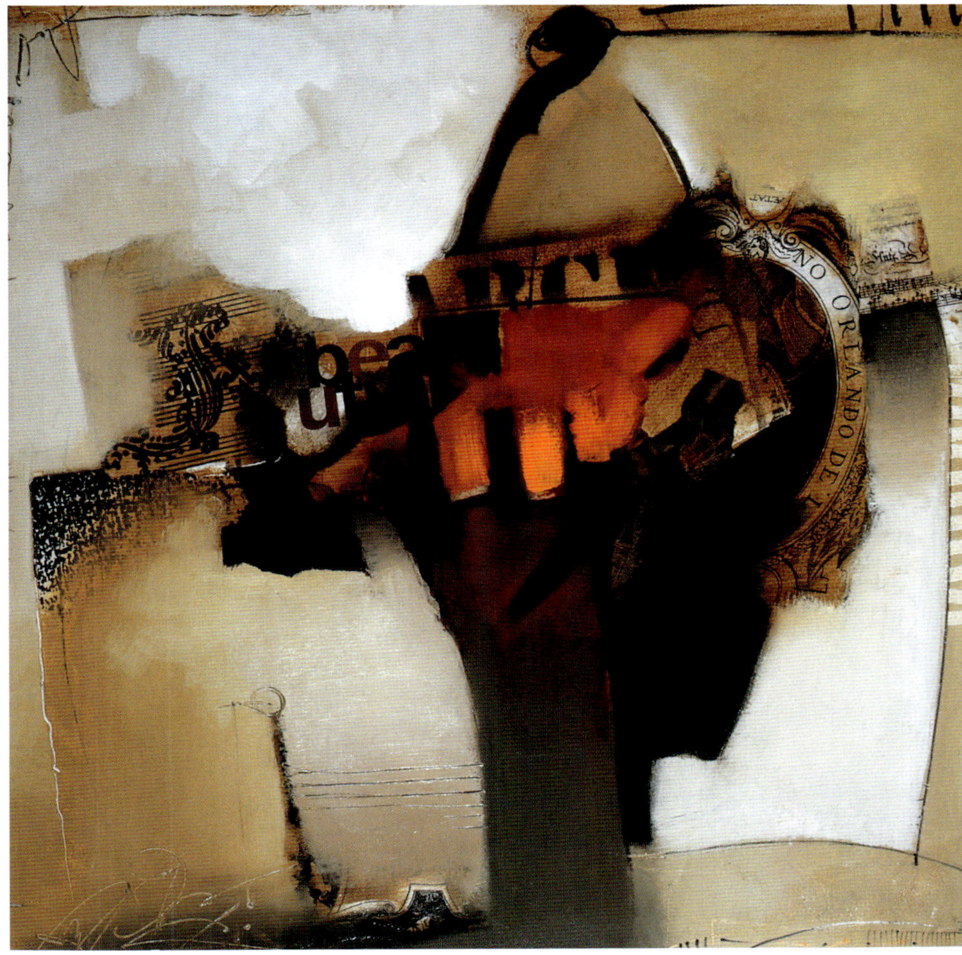

images wild, the Virgin, child."

William Blake

The paintings, because of their focus on the contrasting strains of color and form, remind us of the devotional images in both eastern and western art. These contrasting images are also the source of the energies that make the **"Ledger Line"** paintings primal and free. The contrasting meanings evoked by these paintings remind me of a few stanzas by William Blake:

"Seek those images that constitute the wild, the lion and the Virgin, the Harlot and the child."

Melodium
Etude Polonaise I
Mixed Media on Paper 20"x20"

Moreover, these paintings offer us an abstract vision of musical forms and allusions of harmonies. The objects are reduced to their skeletal structures, recognizable only as types, establishing metaphysical principles rather than tangible experiences. **"Ledger Line, Guitar Etude II"**[26] is austere and laconic and, because of this simplicity, it is all encompassing, open to many readings and emotionally powerful.

The shadow of the guitar is as foretelling as are the shadows cast by the women of Munch's paintings. The contrasting of the forms with the void moves us to illusionism and metaphor, where the obscurity and opacity of the painting leave plenty of room for a dance of the fantastic and banal.

At the heart of these works lies the notion of contrast: dark and light, idea and sensation, form and void, motion and rest. **"Guitar Etude III"**[27] is multi-layered as its border functions like a cosmic space into which either enters or shoots out the painted imagery. The distance of void between the center and its frame intensifies feelings by contrasting the outward with the inward manifestations. The **"Guitar Etude"** paintings are themselves musical pieces.

They have managed, in an Orphist vein, to transmute form into sound. The only other painter that I can think of who was successful in this regard was Arthur Dove, a friend of Georgia O'Keeffe and a towering artist in the first half of the twentieth century. Dove's works, like the **"Ledger Line"** paintings of Emanuel, succeeded in communicating the sensations of physical experiences rather than the physical form itself. **"Precis I"**[21] is abstract enough that, if not for its place in the series, it would not have been morphologically identifiable. It is a work whose function is poetic and musical, and therefore open-ended regarding signification and meaning. In these works the issue of artistic interpretation is paramount and the object loses its identity to the artist's emotional center. Here we are closer to Kandinsky's theory of electrical vibrations—emanated by thoughts and feelings and expressed in color and form without any regard for logical-conventional syntax. As musical sources, these works are most successful in transmitting sound and even melody. The **"Ledger Line"** paintings rely more heavily upon subconscious feelings than any other series, including the **"Appellation"** paintings. While these works are not spontaneous enough to be improvisations, they are nevertheless compositionally symbolic and move from reason to feeling, from language to lyricism. In the **"Ledger Line"** paintings, forms are suspended in a void. Weight defers to weightlessness, just as the colors, by highlighting the contrasts, serve as the sole force of harmony in the paintings. These works transform matter to musical energy and evolve into musical release.

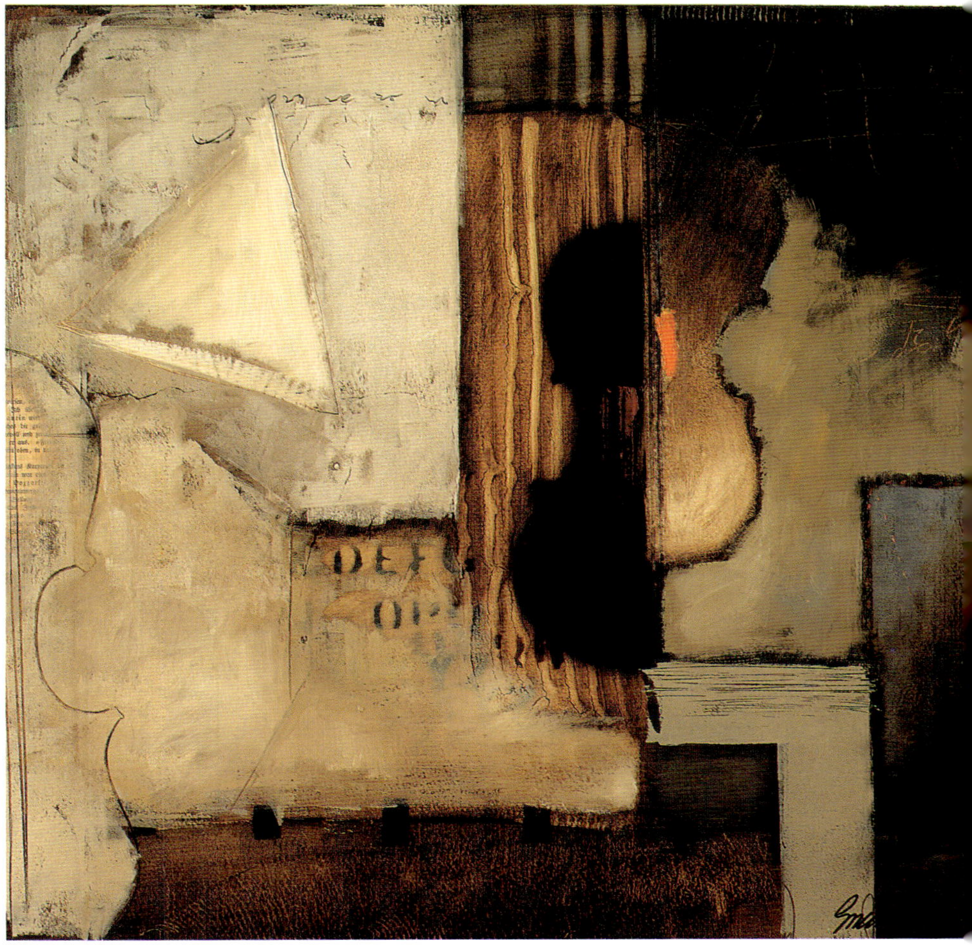

"Melodium"[80-105;113-141] is interesting because it melds classical and contemporary styles. This series also explores variations on the theme of music and its related metaphors. The settings are often landscapes formed in the spirit of collage: candles, medieval manuscripts, columns, chairs, architecture and more are assembled in a softened atmosphere redolent with the genteel quality of chamber music. By contrast, the **"Orchestration"** series is full of hard edges and evokes a far more intellectually ordained sense of composition. Because of its baroque allusions, **"Melodium"** is romantic and evokes a heroic sense of its setting. In **"Melodium"** we are less concerned with the designs of the instruments than we are with the moods they evoke. The setting is clearly the device through which the flesh and spirit of this music is emotionally interpreted. **"Melodium, Incantata"**[86] for example, is congenial to the

Melodium
Solano Fall I

Mixed Media on Paper 20"x20"

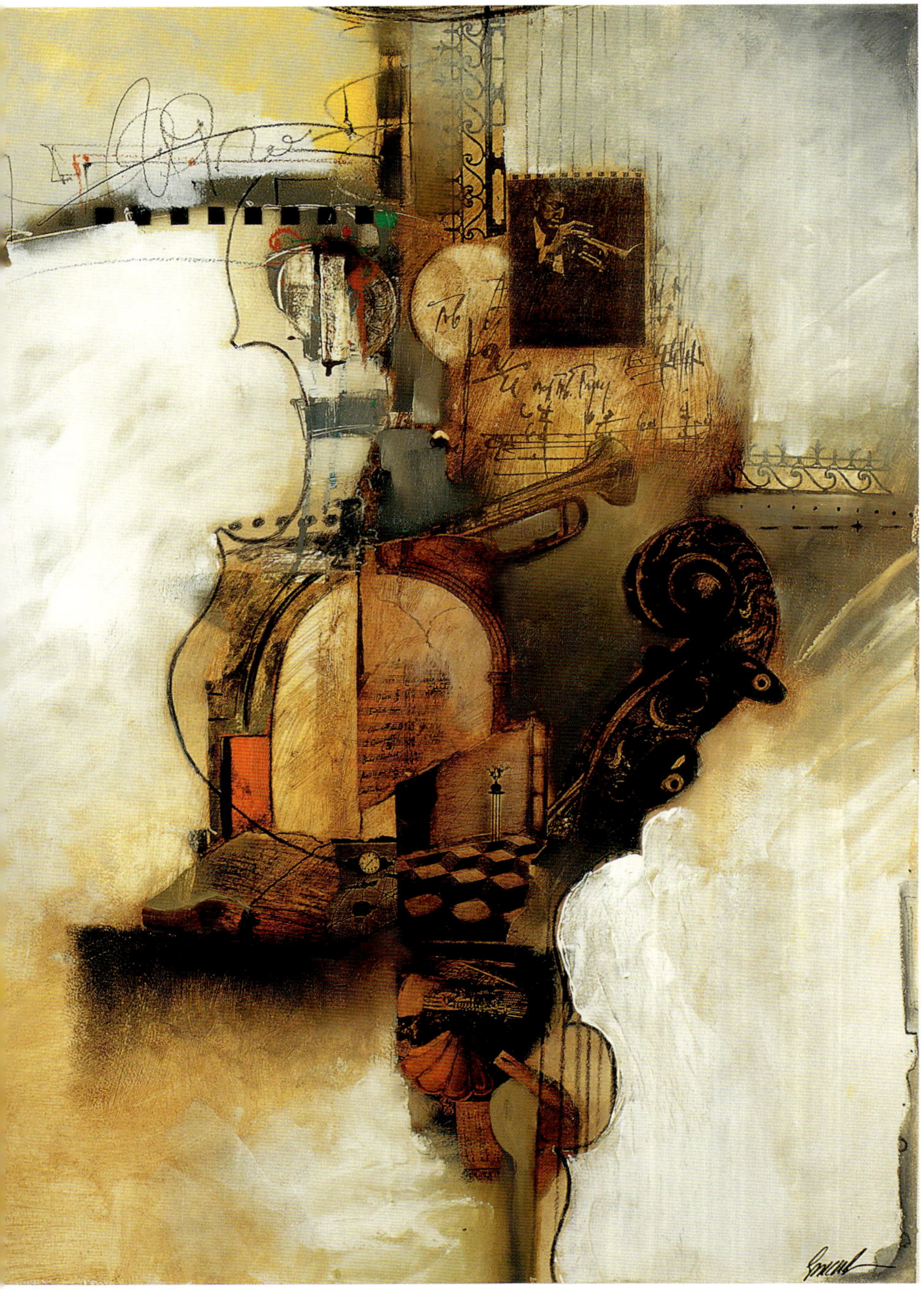

"Only what

ostentatious settings of baroque art. Its rich environment is drenched with a light beyond the candles and evokes an otherness that may be viewed as spiritual, visionary and ideal. The golden space that defines most of the settings in this series of paintings sweeps us upward into its mysteries with the musical instruments as seraphic forms, alluding to some otherworldliness.

Emanuel arrives at abstraction with a variety of forms and techniques. Collage is one of his most effective methods of changing reality into transcendental issues. In most of his works, be they **"Orchestration," "Ledger Line"** or **"Passages[55-57],"** the effect is collage-like, even if the collage technique is not utilized. The truncated and fragmentary forms arranged at random decontextualize the objects and deprive them of their conventional signification. In fact, they easily remind us of the French poet Mallarmé, whose comments about language are quite relevant and related to the visual collage. Mallarmé wrote: "They are the same words that the bourgeois reads every morning—the very same! But then (and here his smile broadened), if he finds them again in one of my poems he no longer understands them! That's because they have been rewritten by a poet."

Like Mallarmé, at the heart of Emanuel's images is a desire to avoid repetition of older ideas and phrases. His collages move us beyond the shopworn meanings and into new notations and arrangements. Given that the new meanings are now fully subjective, then innumerable values arise, making for a very rich picture of ideas and sensations.

can be seen there is there." Frank Stella

More needs to be said about his collage-like arrangements where forms burst forth with energies that revolve into their neighboring spaces. These arrangements, though modern and subjective, are nevertheless baroque in their amplitude and corporeality. The massive forms create an impression of a choir with giant musical pillars leading to both passion and enigma. This space also allows for the images to create energies in multiple directions and amplify the energies of the instruments' implied tonalities. It would be a mistake to read these forms only in physical terms and to ignore their transubstantiative powers; the baroque amplitude of these paintings evokes the presence of a chorus leading us to a crescendo. Furthermore, this arrangement is a device for heightening intellectual ambiguity and giving free reign to lyricism. In addition, the sizes and the shapes of the **"Orchestration"** canvases allow for artful release and constraint. The vertical frames of **"Orchestration XII"**[64] and **"XI"**[65] create a sense of claustrophobia while the horizontal frames allow for release and catharsis.

Form and Anti-form

In Emanuel's later abstractions, the forms of **"Orchestration"** and **"Concerto"** dissolve into shadowy morphologies, losing any semblance of their objective selves as they change into counterpoints of dark and light. Recognizable forms rapidly give way to organic-gestural abstractions and color field paintings, making for a theatre of birth and death and a metamorphosis of space into matter. In these works, the contrast of mass and void and, indeed, the oppositions created by their shapes, move beyond the **"Ledger Line"** paintings and thus generate quantum energies. Emanuel's amorphous abstractions are

Mixed Media on Canvas 40"x54"

imaginative peregrinations into genesis and loss, creation and silence as forms appear and rapidly mutate away from themselves. This is especially true of **"Epilogue I"**[143] where the images and colors suggest an embryonic state of metamorphic process. What appear as alien fields of color and energies penetrate into one another, while also resisting full absorption and, thus, unity. Here and there a recognizable image appears like an avatar of Visnu the Creator only to be changed into some ineffable and inexplicable presence by the shamanistic magic of the moving forms. Mallarmé defined art as "hyperbolic," meaning that a great work transcends its own conditions of creation and appears to be self-created. **"Hyperbole I"**[149] is one of those paintings: a soft and gentle confrontation of forms and colors is also cataclysmic. The silences of its spaces are also shrieks when seen in their confrontational lights. In this context, Ad Reinhardt's comment that "you can only make absolute statements negatively" is appropriate, for the dark and lighter spaces are in extremes. The hidden and the revealed are in both forms and colors. When art is protected from its creator, when it exists without any connection to he who claims a genetic right to it, then it is the mysterious spiritual place in which we all dwell. This painting, more so than any other of his abstractions illustrated in this essay, fits Mallarmé's definition of "hyperbolic," for it is a metaphysical occurrence articulating its own spirituality rather than the hands that have created it.

Some of Emanuel's paintings remind me of the works of one of the greatest, and clearly one of the fathers of postmodern art, Joseph Beuys. Beuys, who saw himself as a Shaman and believed in art's alchemical powers, saw forms as suggestive of truths that rationality could not access. **"Epilogue I"**[143] and **"Hyperbole I"**[149] are in many ways alchemical processes of change and everlasting mutation. They are reminiscent of Beuys' spiritual paintings, where what we confront is a symbolic pregnancy alluding to infinite perceptions that are intuitive and spiritual rather than empirical. Theodore Adorno wrote that, "The more spiritual the works of art are, the more they erode their substance." And, indeed, the simplicity of these substances exists in the most complex of assemblies. The voids and silences of **"Hyperbole I"**[149] are not nihilistic but creative, as they set the stage for possibilities. For, in these gestural expressions, voids are also that which the French artist Jean Arp called "concrete forms." In these paintings, each act of dematerialization serves as a new, unique and non-iterate materialized vision. They do not negate existence but affirm a form of transcendental spirituality which the rational and the empirical world cannot possibly embody.

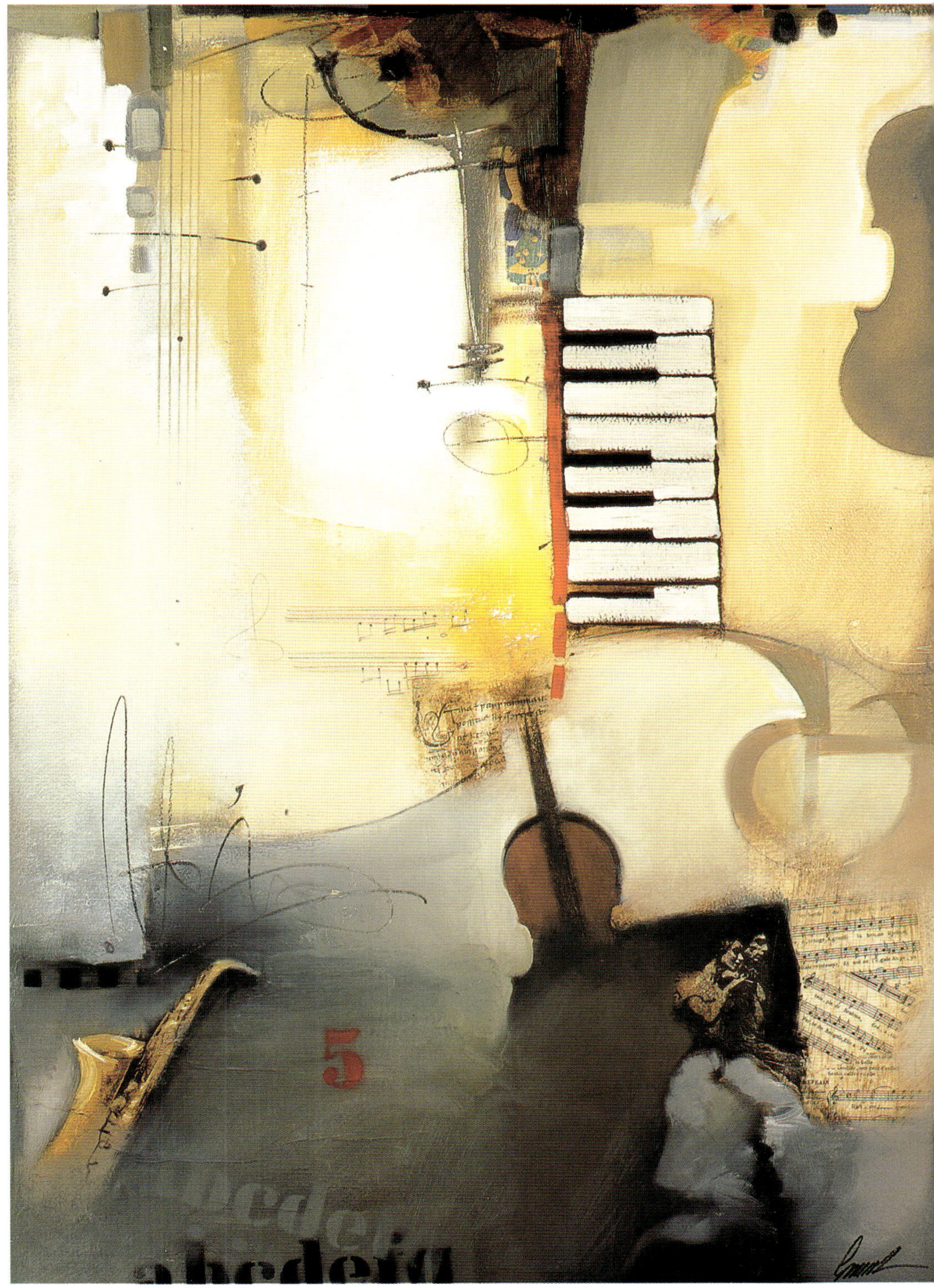

Self-sufficiency and Insufficiency of Art

Modernists such as Henri Matisse believed in the self-sufficiency of art while the Postmodernists, as exemplified by the deconstructivist works of Chris Burden, point to the insufficiency of art. For Matisse, as for Mallarmé, a genuine artistic expression, when sprung from an individuated center, was complete and withstood the scrutiny of time. In Postmodernism, on the other hand, one cannot with certainty define either a genuine expression or individuality. It seems that at the end of the century we have recognized the failings of our brave modernist beginnings. The artist as the original creator is now replaced with the artist as a creation of the critic. Art as a sensational reflection is now art as the madness of art. Nothing promised by Modernism has come to pass and a disappointed generation of artists have taken to alien and strange ways to discover themselves elsewhere and as others. Political unrest in the second half of the century has not helped matters either. Artists affected by wars, political and religious fanaticism, have found themselves in diaspora crisscrossing the globe searching for an artistic home. In so doing they have carried aspects of their own cultures and assimilated them in their new homes and vice versa.

Moreover, the information age has furthered the exchange of cultural traits and has hastened the end of any meaningful distinctions in any culture's art. Art is now a matter of juxtapositions and the manner of its juxtaposing reveals something about the nature of our being in this time and place. As different cultural traits and different spirits assimilate art, the end product, because of its contradictions and antinomies, can no longer claim self-sufficiency. It stands suspended between cultures and expressive zones.

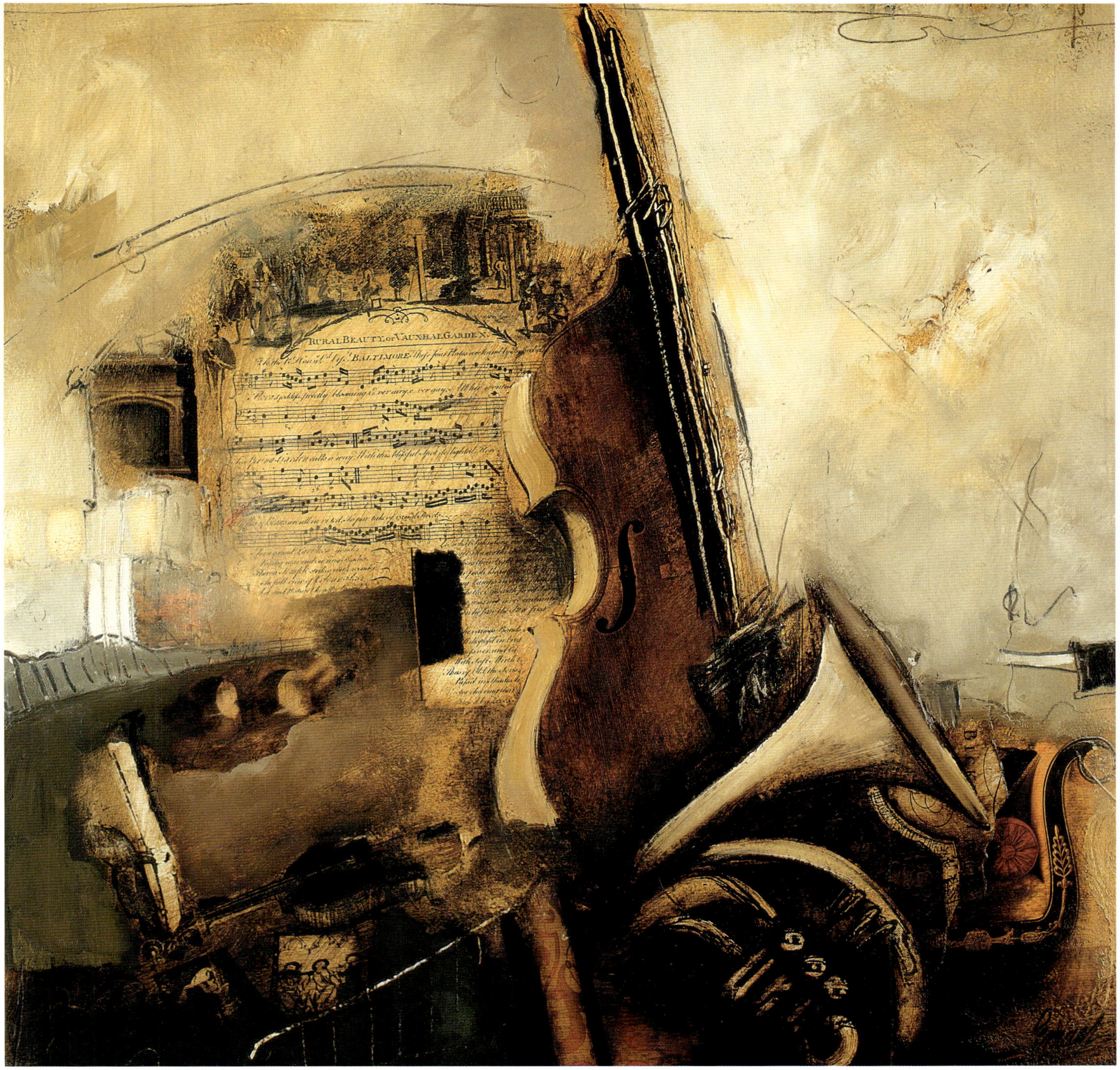

Melodium
Memoir III

Mixed Media on Paper 20"x20"

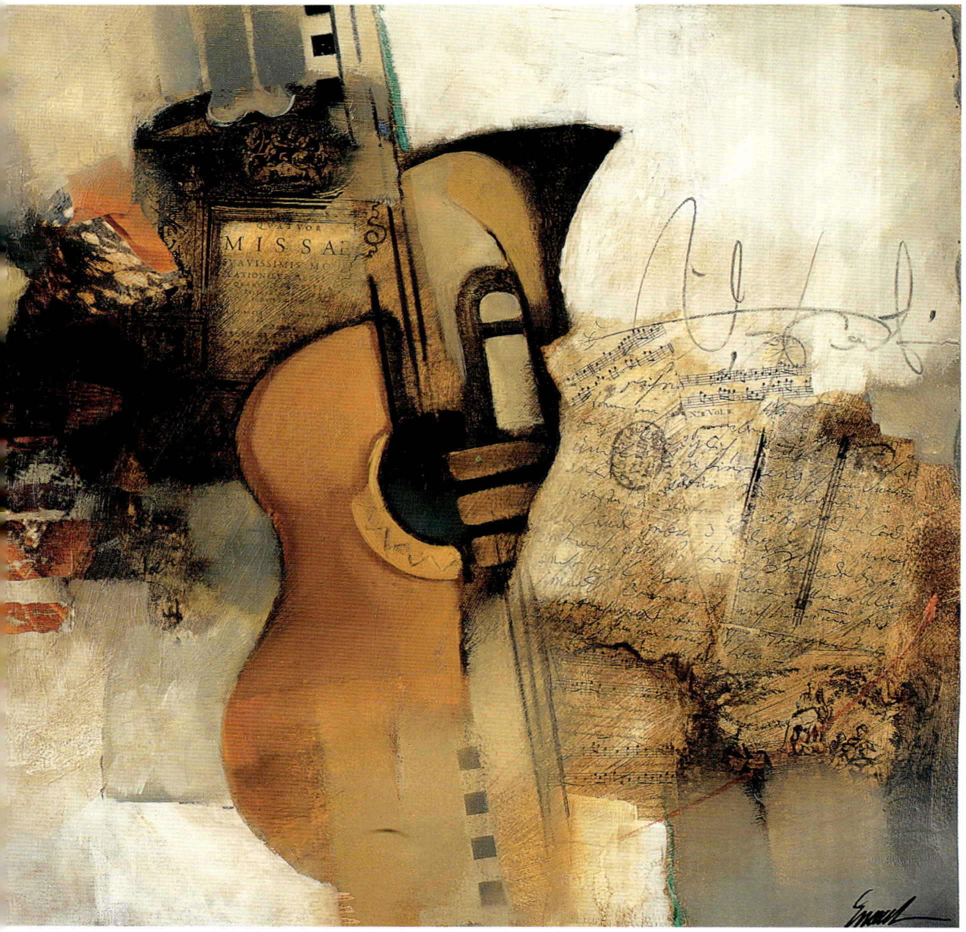

The new art's melting pot now looks at decorative patterns and compositions that are not western in origin. Artists such as Miriam Schapiro and Joyce Kozloff, among many others, are as inspired by middle eastern and far eastern designs and compositions as they are by their own native traditions. The Metropolitan Museum of Art's exhibition of Persian manuscript painting, "A King's Book of Kings: The Shahnameh of Shah Tahmasp" and "Tagasode," a show of Japanese kimonos are two of the many non-western art shows often cited as major sources of design for some postmodern artists. Kozloff's repertoire, for example, includes Persian, Japanese, French and Coptic motifs. Emanuel is truly at home in this postmodern context. **His complexity is partly motivated by the multi-cultural portraits that belie his art.**

Babak Emanuel was born in Shiraz, Iran. Shiraz's fame as a city of arts and music is well known and to this day its past glories occupy a major chapter of Iranian history and artistic traditions. The legend of Shiraz claims that many of its inhabitants are deeply influenced by its creative past. If so, the impact of Shiraz may be seen obliquely and indirectly as an emotional infrastructure in Emanuel's fascination with themes of nostalgia and music. His poetic phrasing, especially in **"Hallycon,"**[6;14-15] which is laden with sighs, fragrance and even sorrow, has a baroque quality with only its psychological roots linked to Emanuel's native land. Likewise, the taut mannerist images of **"Casa,"**[6;16-17] with its gothic proportions alluding to incommensurability, are emotional traits of Iranian art, while their physical substantiations are purely western.

Mixed Media on Paper 20"x20"

Melodium

Emanuel left Iran in 1983 and upon arriving in Atlanta became immersed in the arts. In America, the paintings of Motherwell, Tapis and Rauschenberg had the greatest impact upon his aesthetic sensibilities. Traces of Motherwell are still present in his abstractions and collages. As Robert Hughes said, "Before it is anything else, collage is play. The rules of the game are subsumed in what is the mailing paper, matchboxes, cigarette packs, chocolate wrappers, stickers and other stuff in the unstable flux of messages and signs that pass through a painter's studio." And Emanuel's collages are indeed playful. However, his collages, as depicted in **"Passages"**, move beyond the western oeuvres portrayed by Braque and Motherwell. This series dissembles within its forms a lugubrious romanticism which contrasts with the fully transcendent games played by Motherwell and Braque. The **"Passages"** series evokes a mood of nostalgia and a pre-sentiment for longing. The past hovers and haunts the spaces of each of these works. The present moment is only for wistful ruminations and cannot be fully liberated from the objective world, from language and therefore from memory. In these paintings, ochre colored arches serve as windows to intimate worlds that are filled with romantic flourishes. **"Memorabilia II"**[56] with its old photographs and antiquated buildings, conveys the psychological intricacies of remembrance. I have no doubt that in this juxtaposition of abstract forms and Romanticism is a combination of the eastern psyche and the western syntax.

In fact, a glance at Emanuel's paintings reveals a dialectical structure that melds a wide range of styles and aesthetic experiences: Modernism, Postmodernism, Baroque and Romanticism and, even though concealed beneath his fully contemporary imagery, eastern art. **"Concerto"** and **"Melodium"** are two examples of such a perspective. In **"Melodium"** a modernist vision of forms and designs is given an extravagant baroque and neo-classical setting. The paintings of **"Concerto"** likewise transport the modern musical forms, with their golden backgrounds, into religious icons. At all times the artistic foundations of Emanuel's paintings and the symbolic formulations of his shapes reveal a conflation of energies that are, to some degree, paradigmatic of the oppositions between Transcendentalism, Romanticism and Western Abstraction. These issues are fully manifest in his various series covering different styles and emotional visions.

His art is, therefore, as in the works of Kozloff and Schapiro, touched by historical experiences that are at times unaccommodating. But if the worlds portrayed seem irreconcilable, it is because the realities of the contemporary world are also irreconcilable. And it is this irreconcilability that has made the lexicon of postmodern art so synthetic, thus always alluding to some insufficiency that requires regression and re-examination of our past selves. As in Sartre's **Nausea**, the systems of knowledge that have defined the world are no longer sufficient for sorting and understanding its elements. One cannot help but conclude that the arbitrary juxtapositions of these borrowed elements allude to some temporal disorder where the linear and the orderly progression of thoughts and events are replaced with chaos. It is this issue that makes the reading of Emanuel's paintings, or other post-modern works, labyrinthine and also exciting.

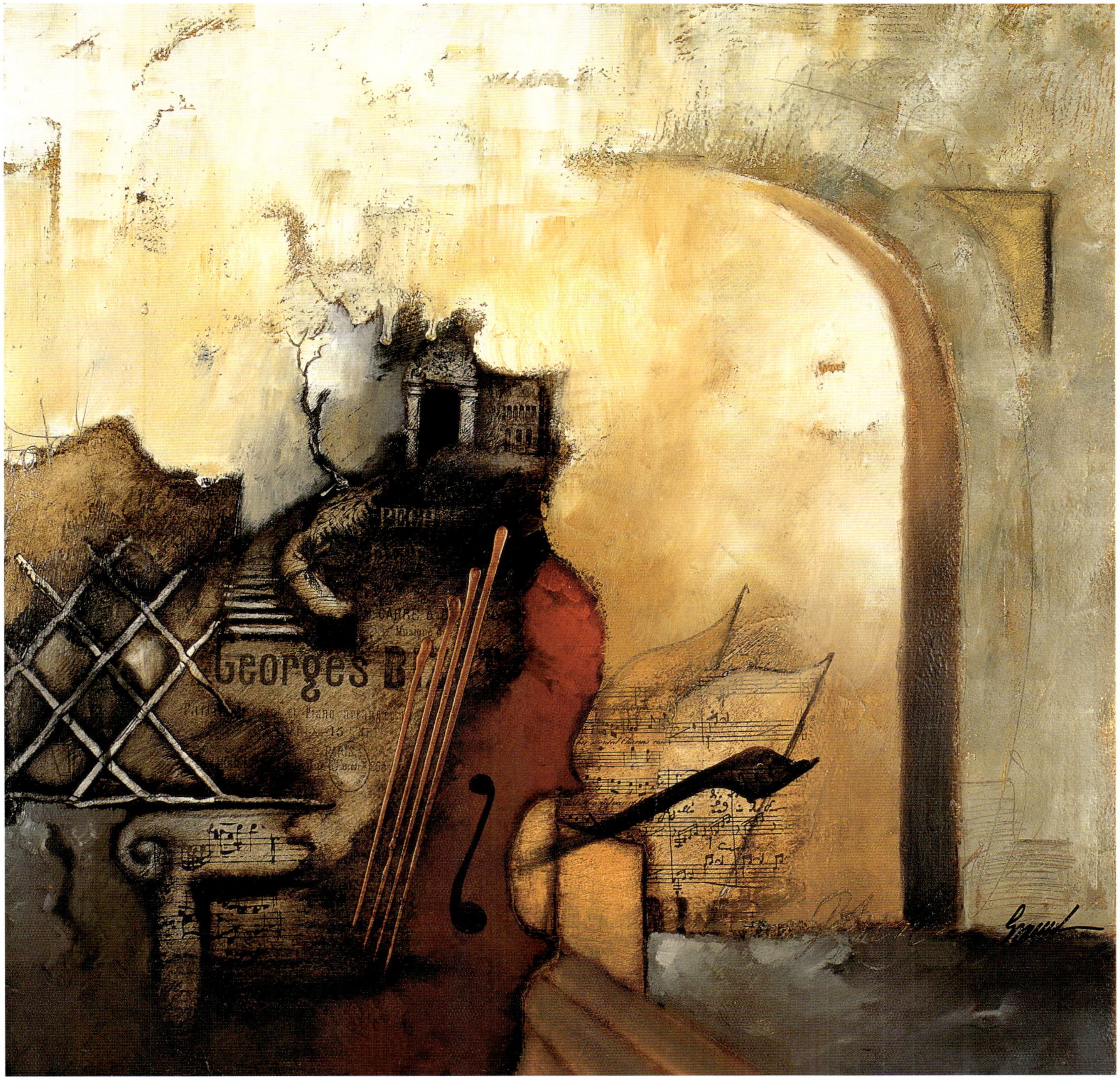

Melodium
Metaphor & Memory II

Mixed Media on Paper 20"x20"

As I have already mentioned, the interzonal qualities of **"Melodium," "Concerto"** and **"Hallycon"** may in part be explained by the dissolution of cultural borders and also by the technological advances that have transformed the globe into a village. But to a great extent they are also due to the epistemological breakdowns that have defined the last quarter of the twentieth century. One dimension of this breakdown in our systems of knowledge is expressed in terms of integrated morphologies, the likes of which Emanuel's art so powerfully exemplifies. **"Melodium,"** for example, reminds us partly of the "grand style" of baroque and partly of modern accents. These images, as in **"Passages,"** draw upon the baroque anatomies of passion on the one hand, and distinguish themselves on the other hand, by reticent and formal scales of modern art. This trait, appearing in all media, including architecture, literature and music, has produced a pneumonic art and, unlike Modernism, allows for memory to be a constant presence in its expressions. Therefore, unlike Modernism, the artist does not express his primal and unadulterated confrontation with the world, but returns to history and re-interprets its many extant faces.

The regressive proclivities in postmodern art, though scanty and desultory in their focus, have brought back so much of a past that Modernists had either ignored or discarded. Now many Postmodernists, be they Robert Mappelthorpe, Dan Douke or Robert Venturi, allow the past to flow through their conscious or subconscious minds, but in unpredictable ways and patterns. One of Emanuel's series that best exemplifies this trait is **"Hallycon."** The paintings of this series, like the the works of Cindy Sherman revisiting the paintings of Caravaggio, or Louise Lawler reproducing Andy Warhol's images, are a play on the presences and absences of history. These works convey in one regard, the perseverance of history and, in another regard, the adulteration of the transmission of historical facts because of the many intermediaries that are always present, i.e. the personality of the artist, the context of its appearance and the state of interpretation at the time of its reading.

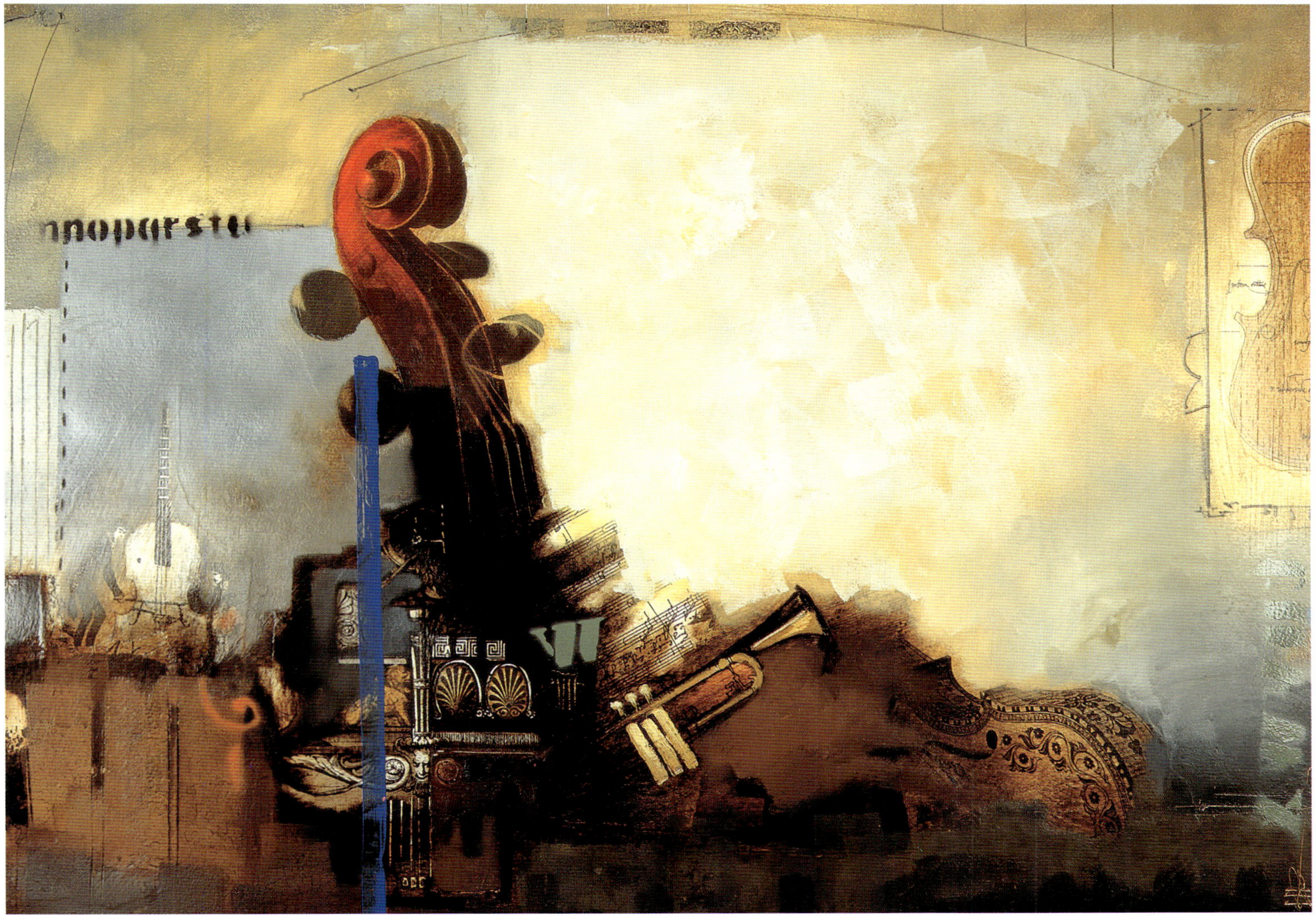

Melodium Lyrica I

Mixed Media on Paper | 34"x24"

"Hallycon," as a series, distinguishes itself by being idiomatic of classical and modern, conscious and subconscious, reality and dream. These paintings occupy an aesthetic niche of their own and remind me of the works of John Swihart, where the past is reinterpreted in a contemporary light. The emotional theatre of Halcyon vaguely fits the realities of the world, for the element of subconscious, and thus the inscrutable, in these paintings is ever present. In each of the **"Hallycon"** paintings there is an allusion to the principle of spiritual and physical elevation by making references to bygone styles and sensibilities which sweep us upward and beyond.

In **"Hallycon,"** the darker tones ebb and flow with a spiritual voice that is evoked by its icon-like colorings. They are poetic visions contrasting the serenity of the settings with the psychological charge of their colors. In these works, with the luminescence of gems, Emanuel paints landscapes of intimate, idealized rural scenes. Rolling hills and colorful trees vibrate with the energies of time-effaced paint which claim roots in past histories and experiences. The unpopulated one-lane roads of these paintings snake gracefully into a horizon framed by brooding, ancient skies. The roads amplify the sense of mystery lurking at the heart of these forms and colors. The deep, rich colors, juxtaposing dark, mossy green against umber and rust tones, coupled with silhouettes of trees, lead us to a familiar but unknown dimension contrasted against the open, crackled skies. The skies are instrumental in setting the mood by capturing the colors and textures of ancient Roman and Christian frescoes. Umber mixes with various gray tones to add warmth and the illusion of aging, which is sometimes further enhanced by the crackled skies as seen in **"Hallycon IV"**[6] and **"Hallycon VII."**[14]

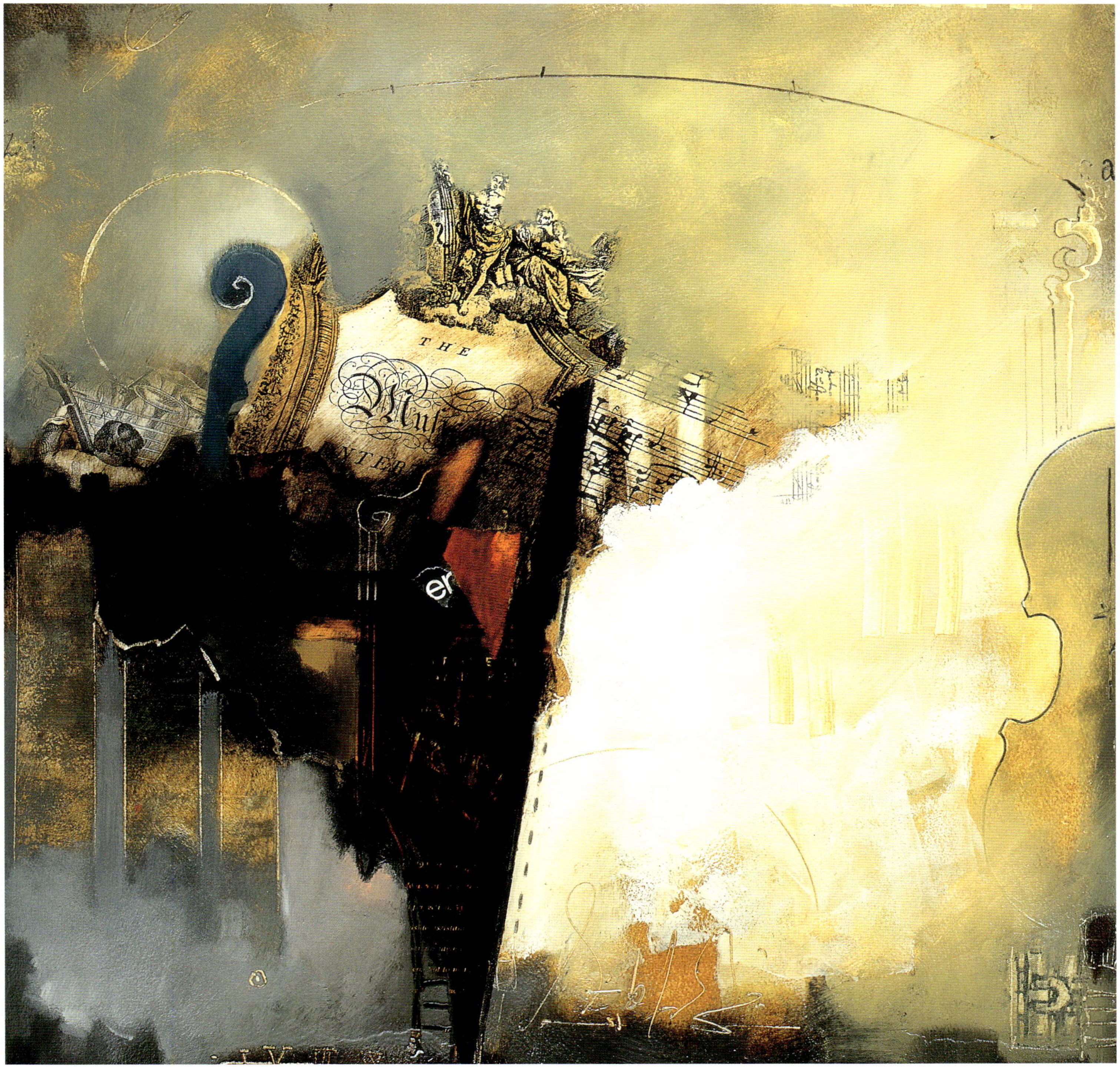

Melodium Lyrica II

Mixed Media on Paper 20"x20"

The complexity of lighting, which seems to emanate from within the forms, creates a sense of the spiritual found only in the sacred art of the Middle Ages and the icons of Christian art. The absence of detail in these paintings, less concerned with reality than with mood, further enhances their sensational effect. The darker and antiquated colors exude a nervous energy that is fitting of the mannerist paintings. Had the tones corresponded to natural colors, so much of the spiritual and iconic impact would have been lost. The **"Hallycon"** paintings are placed at the edge of reality and dreams, and vibrate with a mysterious energy—a baroque power that transubstantiates matter into signs which allude to high and transcendent emotions. In other words, the **"Hallycon"** paintings equivocate matter and spirit, and release energies that serve as metaphors of the sublime confronting the awesome.

The **"Hallycon"** paintings are one of the few non-abstract styles of Emanuel. They present a natural perspective with rhythms and measures that are platonic, ideal and harmonious. Being inside of one of these spaces is akin to dreaming of truths that wakeful moments refuse to acknowledge. The momentum created by the vigor of its coloring is enthralling in the sense that it transports us to the twilight of realization before language had corrupted essence.

The paintings of **"Hallycon"** also allude to critical theoretical issues that are at the heart of both Modernism and Postmodernism. Modernism had fully removed itself from history and tradition, thus giving abstraction the voice that declared history anachronistic. The artists of Modernism, consciously or subconsciously, rejected the past, believing that art could be original and primal without a trace of the past. Postmodernism on the other hand regresses into traditional structures, capsizing the most sacred dictum of the modern age: originality or creation out of a primal ground. Picasso and Miró, for example, believed that they could see and paint as children; namely, free of memory and language. Or for Vlaminck and Boccioni, among many others, history was erasable. As the critic Clement Greenberg said, the modern artist, "in search of the absolute...tries in effect to imitate God by creating something valid solely on its own terms...content to be dissolved so completely into form that the work of art or literature cannot be reduced in whole or in part to anything not itself." The postmodern dictum is, on the other hand, about referencing a work of art or literature to something other than itself. In **"Hallycon,"** as in Nabokov's **Lolita** or Faulkner's **Light in August,** we see art show its dependence on earlier narratives and its propensity to sustain itself by their lingering memories. In this regard, the Byzantine and iconic qualities of **"Hallycon"** dramatically wrench the accents of a world that conveys an astonishing sense of complicity with history and its narratives. Thus the **"Hallycon"** paintings make commentaries on how the past and present are mysteriously fused by memory. All things return, though not in whole, to some other thing, but not to themselves. And as they are destined to a cycle of eternal referencing, then the reality that they evoke is more a function of interpretation than the recognition of concrete empirical phenomena. Moreover, **"Hallycon"** suggests that material reality, due to the interference of media in transmission, is above all ambiguous, both in form and meaning. In other words, we know the truth of life by regression and not by unadulterated empirical observation. Because of these ambiguities, the paintings are open fields of interpretation or open works releasing energies in many directions: subjective and objective; prophetic and quotidian.

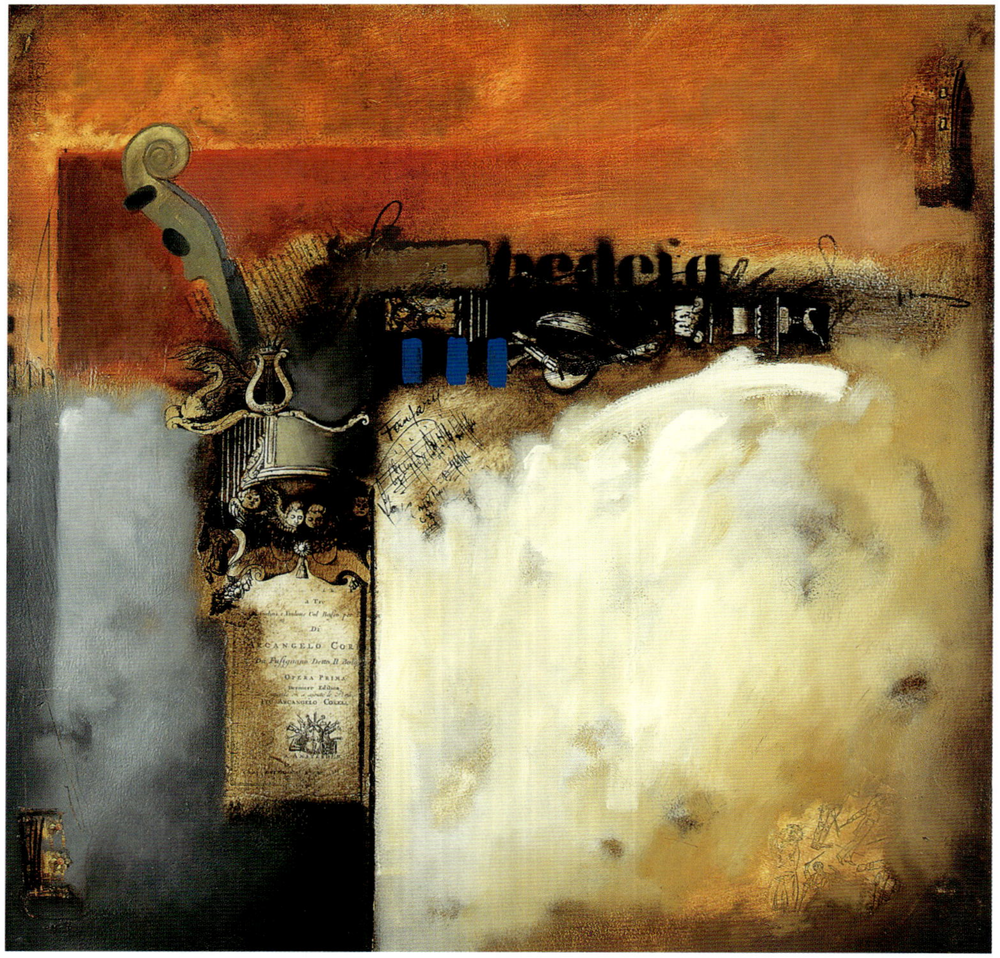

"Hallycon" takes us into magical worlds that lie beyond ourselves. These qualities contrast sharply with **"Orchestration,"** whose abstract and linguistically dissociative compositions are antipodal to the romantic and pastoral expressions of the **"Hallycon"** series. The collage-like juxtapositions of **"Orchestration"** transcend all tangible contexts and abstract the musical objects both spatially and temporally. The same is true of the **"Concerto"** series which, though its setting is dream-like and ephemeral, nevertheless, as in **"Orchestration"** and **"Ledger Line,"** evokes a nominalist sense of signifying. These series, compared to **"Hallycon,"** are less emotional and far more concerned with compositional and intellectual schemes, as the works of Braque before 1918. Similarly, while **"Orchestration," "Concerto"** and **"Ledger Line"** show the abstraction of experience, **"Hallycon"** gives rise to a sense of material palpability that relates to emotional experiences and their moods.

Melodium Lyrica III

Mixed Media on Paper 30"x30"

"I realized early on that artifice attracted me to an image more than any other quality... in the sense of **staging, heightened color and exaggerated lighting**, not a surreal or fictive moment."

Laurie Simmons

"In the **absence** everything became

Art, Memory and Discourse

Artifice is a persistent feature of postmodern art. Primarily, it appears as a response to modernist elitism. Postmodern artifice is politically tendentious and addresses the failings of Modernism. Postmodern artists and writers endowed with cultural and artistic sophistication reveal, as in the photographs of Sherman and the literature of Manuel Puig, the contradictions and artistic displacements of Modernism. We must recognize that the absence of a center in Modernism created a world of individuated values and, thus, interpretations. Nietzsche, who called this condition nihilistic, stressed the demise of metaphysical values, taste and qualitative judgement. Therefore, in a vast and non-centered field of art production, Modernists set out to undermine distinctions and epistemic evaluations. Yet, despite their intent, the opposite occurred and Modernism promoted an elitist view of art and architecture that was, and still is, exclusive in its tastes. In response, Postmodernism, either by design or inadvertently, has tried to overcome the exclusivity of modernist aesthetics by resurfacing all that Modernism had denied and rejected.

of a center or origin
discourse."

David
Lehman

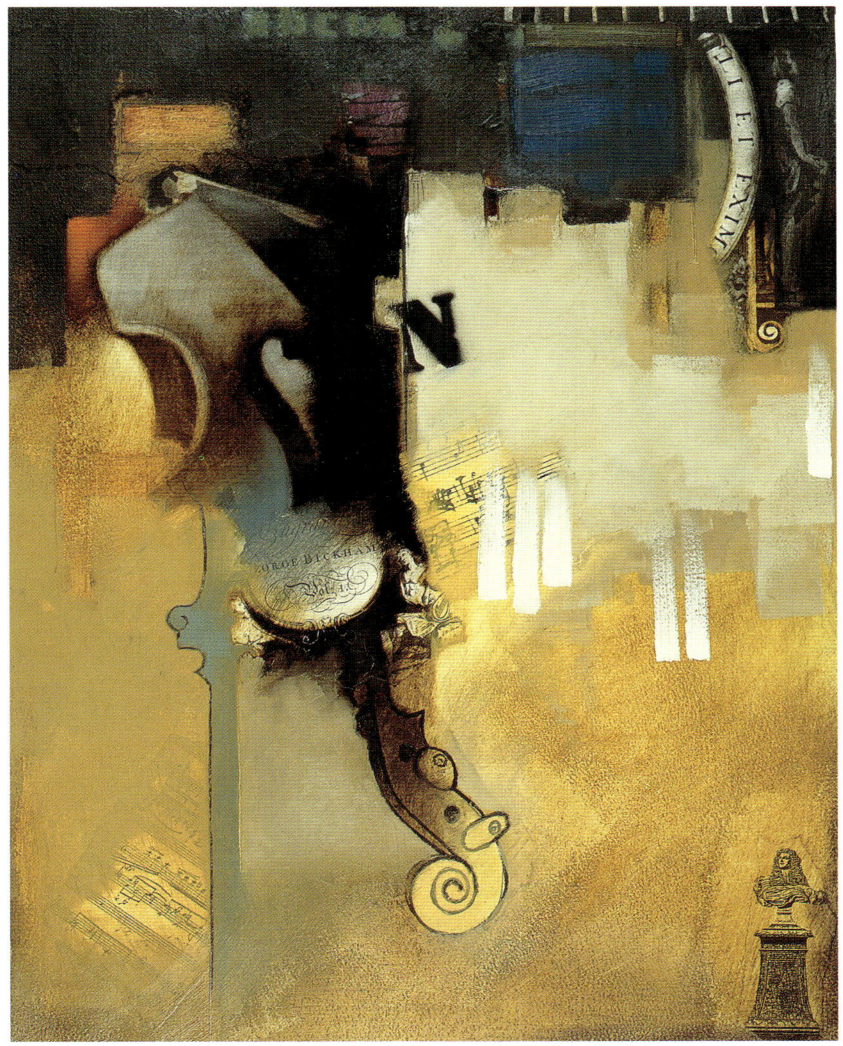

Melodium
Lyrica IV

Mixed Media on Paper 18"x24"

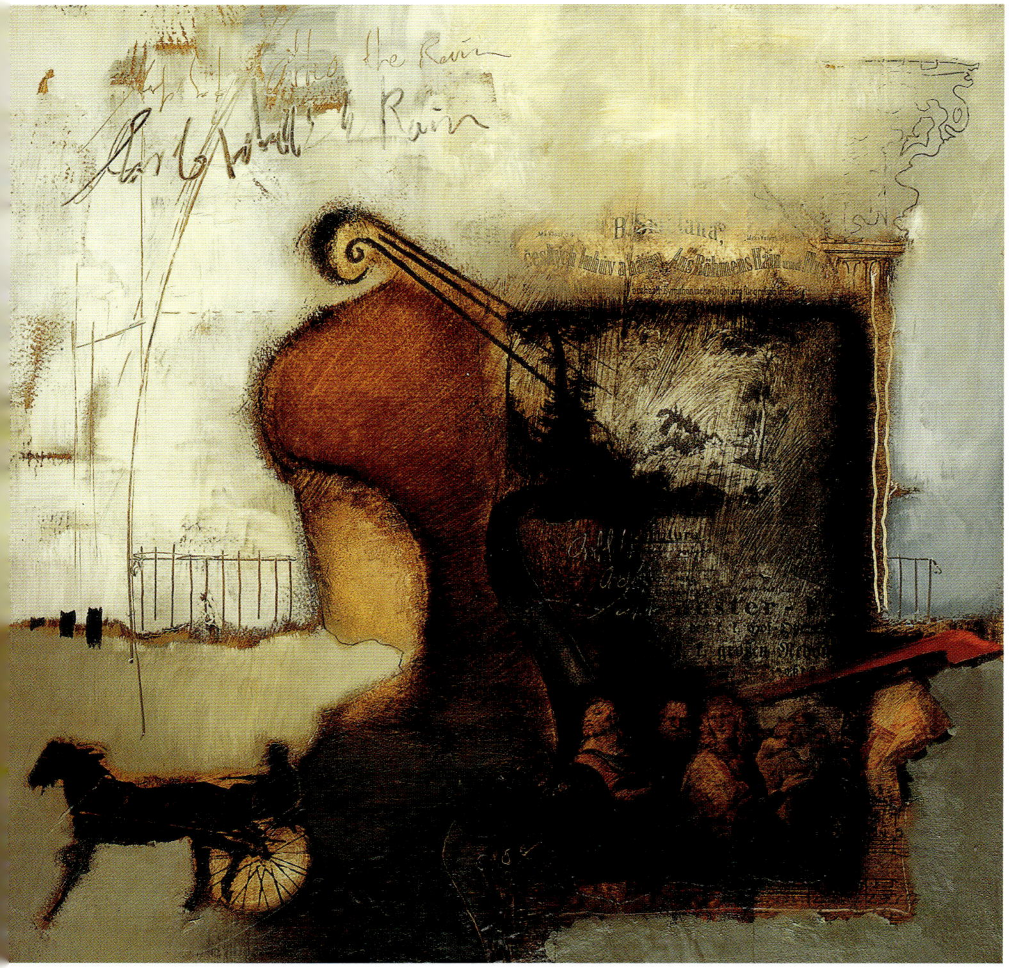

Thus, Postmodernism brings back the art of many economic and aesthetic levels that, though kitsch, are nevertheless one dimension of the West's cultural existence. To give an example, Jeff Koons, in response to this elitism, selects images and artifacts that reveal one ignored dimension of modern life. Therefore, for many postmodern artists artifice is a way of exposing the hidden worlds. Laurie Simmons, Jeff Koons, Cindy Sherman and a host of other artists use artifice to direct our attention to a reality that modern art found unacceptable. Emanuel's **"Casa,"** similar to Koons, uses artifice to resurrect a kitsch that portrayed the tastes and outlooks of a generation in the eighties. Artifice is, for these artists, a consciousness of an idealized style or a stratagem that has turned decorative. Artifice is a statement to remind us of our innate and cultural proclivities to allow the essence to be replaced with appearance as the measure of value.

In addition, artifice also signals a need for referencing. Historical references such as crackling surfaces and classical columns take us back to established signs and symbols that serve as conventional keys to understanding. In **"Passages,"** for example, the references to aged photos, ruins and classical volutes submit to a presentiment for longing and nostalgia as often seen in romantic narratives. Decorum and stagecraft work to release psychological intricacies on wistful reflection and remembrance. The **"Hallycon"** paintings, for example, evoke through romantic flourishes and fashionable images moods and ideas that reference a late medieval

Melodium Lyrica V

Mixed Media on Paper 20"x20"

sense of mystery and sublime realizations. In such a context, artifice is also a secure and grounded language in the face of contemporary breakdowns in communication. By returning to familiar signs, art and language find a haven in the midst of the storms of uncertainty. Often, artifice embraces exaggerated gestures to assert its values as truth. For this reason, artifice is often accompanied with excessive decoration, conceit and pretensions of exquisite pedigree.

The problem of interpreting artifice is, as regarded in Jeff Koons' "String of Puppies" from 1988 and Emanuel's **"Casa"** from the 1990s, whether the images are parodies or discoveries of different valuations. It is now only the intention of the artist that can discern a parody from a genuine expression. The question for us remains whether the artist is making a statement of complicated witticism, alluding that the world is small and commensurate, or is he himself truly the world that he reflects. For the reader, the difference between depth and surface is now only a guess, and the meaning ascribed to a work is a function of the grace of the reader.

Method and Approach

Emanuel's paintings are grouped by series and each series explores a certain theme. These themes range from the abstract to objective and from the real to chimerical. One inherent meaning of a series, as seen from Monet and Warhol is that forms are either mutable and change dramatically in time (Monet) or that they are immutable and remain the same across time and space (Warhol). In the former case, which is seen in Emanuel's art, though these changes are subtle, they are nevertheless important enough to signify epistemic uncertainty. They assert that famous dictum by Wittgenstein that the same word has never been used the same way twice. Each representation, as in the **"Ledger Line"** series, while validated by a universal or transcendental model, is nevertheless unique and non-iterate. In each of Emanuel's series, be they **"Melodium,"** or **"Passages"** we recognize that objects are defined by context and mutate in time. These mutations are a function of subjective perception and also of the world. The variations in each of the series' themes give rise to diverse ontologies and evoke multifarious pictures of the same world. They furthermore undermine any epistemological certainty that the universal models may assert. In other words, Emanuel returns to themes which stand for the ideal or transcendental methodologies. However, unlike Warhol who allows for the ideal to remain as a permanent sign, the variations of his themes descend into the ontology of each moment, thus establishing a world of infinite realities.

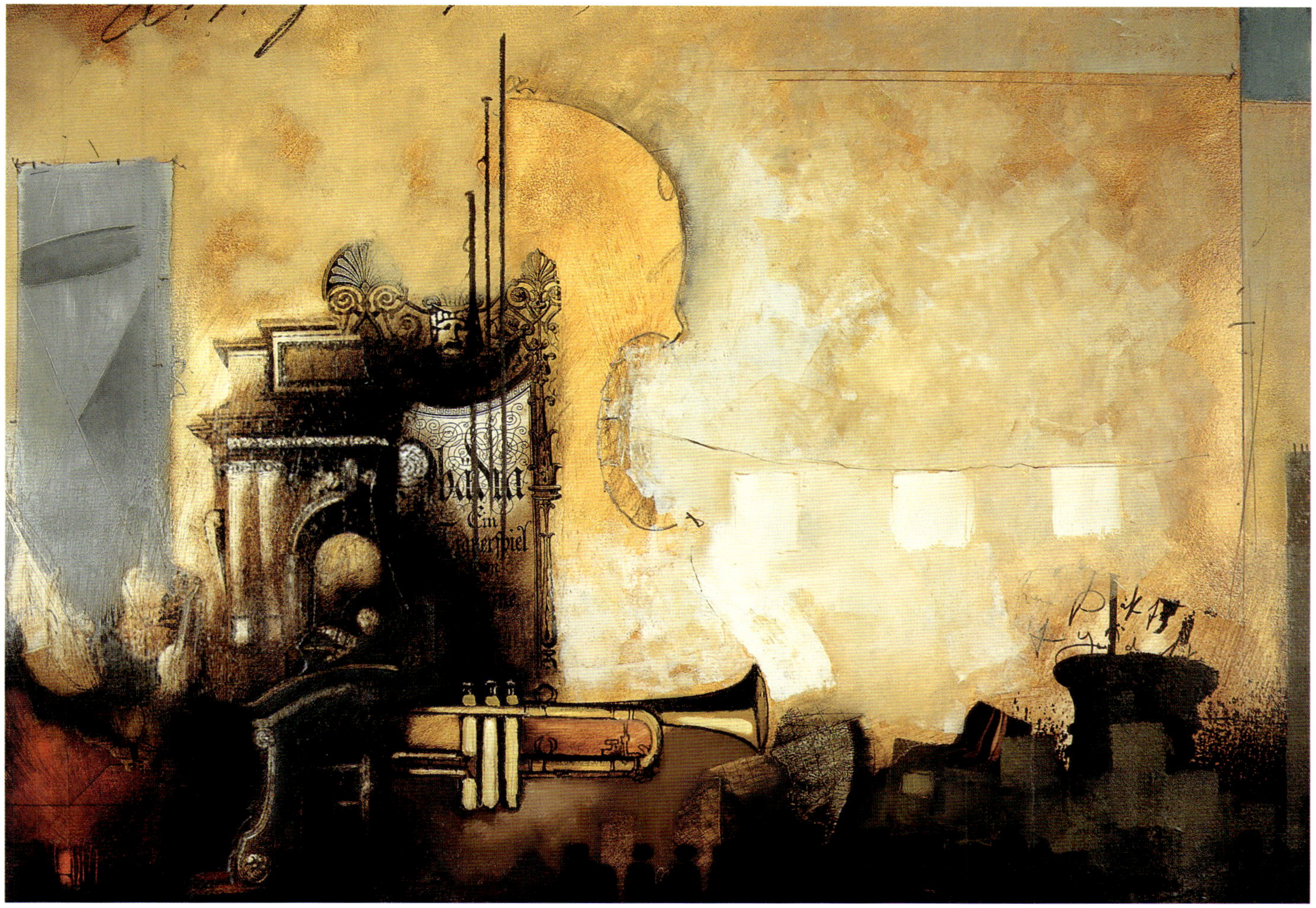

Melodium Lyrica VI

Mixed Media on Paper 34"x24"

Emanuel's various styles refer to a multifaceted picture of a world in transition. Paradoxically, the presence of imagery in **"Hallycon"** establishes rather than transcends the two-dimensionality of the picture plane. The series' painterly approach obscures rather than affirms the reality of the objective forms. The more they allude to the real, the closer we are to recognizing how they have mutated themselves beyond it. **"Hallycon"** differs sharply from the linear and graphic paintings of **"Orchestration"** and **"Passages."** The **"Orchestration"** paintings, for example, make no other claims but to be painted surfaces and, as paintings, they are real. This is partly due to the fact that in the semi-abstract works, and especially in his later mature abstractions exemplified by **"Concerto, Complex Etude II,"**[45] the lines, planes and volumes, while flat, are the three-dimensional world of painting, thus making no pretensions of reproduction or interpretations of reality. His later abstractions arrive at a purist state where paintings are just paintings and no more. In this regard, Frank Stella's famous and oft repeated comment about his paintings that "there is nothing there beside the paint on the canvas" applies to Emanuel's abstract works. His combine paintings, such as **"Concerto, Complex Etude II"**[45] offer us a play on the unmeasured and open spaces of abstractions versus the limited world of objects.

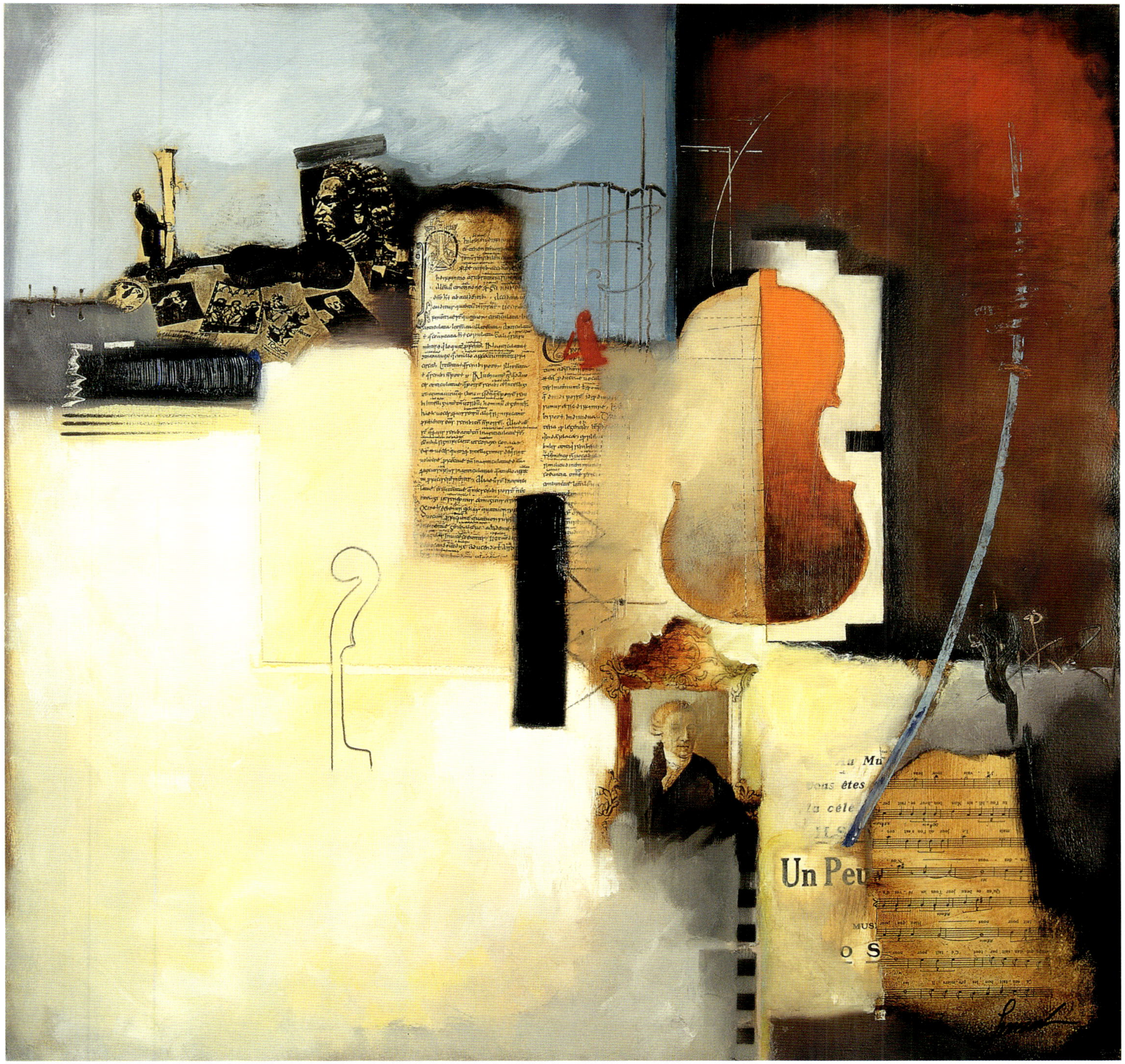

Melodium Lyrica VII

Mixed Media on Paper 30"x30"

The combinations of painterly and linear, open and closed have their precedents in **"Concerto," "Passages"** and **"Melodium."** In his earlier paintings Emanuel combines the open and closed, painterly and linear styles with an order that borders on timidity. In **"Passages,"** for example, the effect of combining the abstract and representational styles is calculated so that one element does not absorb the other. Each style remains within its own confines. In **"Melodium, Lyrica I,"**[127] which is one of the most powerful of his combine paintings, he has become free enough to let the gestural acts define the objective forms. These paintings convey the power of mixing the visceral and emotional. The tactile sensations of **"Melodium, Lyrica I"**[127] are in the recognizable objects, such as the trumpet while the visceral impacts are in the abstract and disembodied designs that engulf them and contextualize the images. The style of these abstractions rejects the romantic over-sensitivity and becomes fully metaphorical.

Many of Emanuel's paintings are suspended somewhere in the transitional spaces of modern and postmodern as well as pop and abstraction. They offer new glimpses into interpretations of collage and beyond—into word-paintings. The use of language concomitant with forms is first seen in **"Passages"** in a manner that reminds us of the modernist collages. Collage uses fragmentary texts and by so doing abstracts the ordinary and the banal object. However, in his later abstract paintings, words appear as independent signs without any connection to some mundane cultural object. In **"Investigation Poetica III,"**[110] the letter S and the numbers 6 and 4 are independent signs and abstract forms in their own right. In his collages, Emanuel would decontexualize a newspaper and thus abstract the object by depriving it of its social and cultural meaning. Here the letters and numbers appear as abstract forms and have morphological content but without a message. Unlike Ed Ruscha's works, writing is not linguistic content, but form and, in this regard, we must compare him to Mallarmé, who saw words not as meanings but as musical sounds.

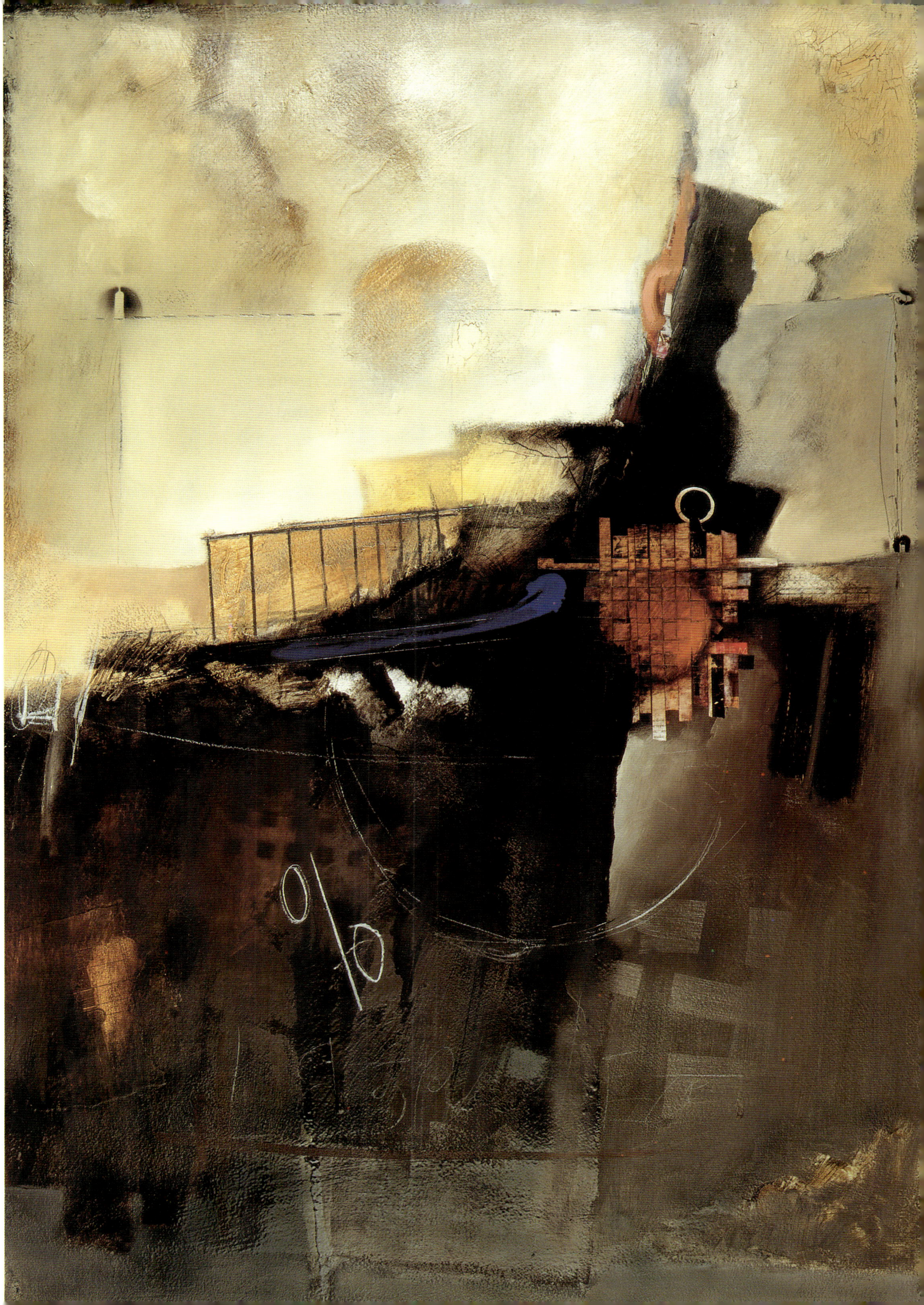

Epilogue I

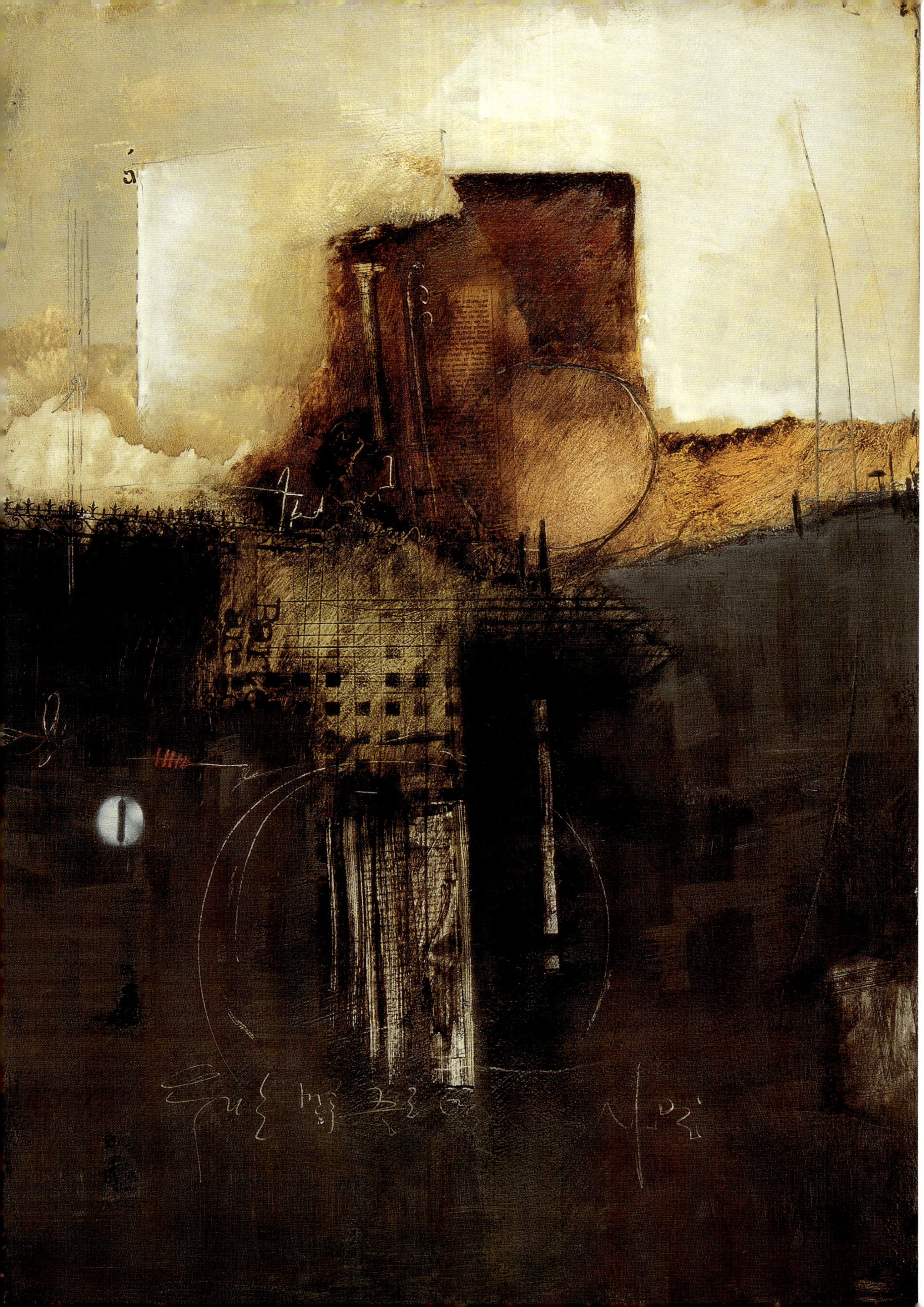

Epilogue II

To go back for a moment to the series of **"Melodium," "Concerto," "Orchestration"** and **"Ledger Line,"** we recognize that Emanuel sought to transcend and abstract through the symbolism of music. Hence, the images of musical instruments served as semiotic references to ideas that are abstract and non-linguistic. I will discuss the significance of music in Emanuel's art later in this essay. For the moment, I would like to show that the structure of these works, especially in **"Concerto," "Ledger Line"** and **"Appellation,"** takes the visible and intelligible signs and carries them by their evocations into opaque and abstract domains. The dominant compositional signature of these paintings is, first and foremost, objective reintegration and then implied abstraction. These paintings are compositionally modern in the sense that they destroy the conventional perspectives and reintegrate the objects of the world in accordance with the artist's solipsism and his sensations.

By contrast, in **"Investigation Poetica III,"**[110] the musical instruments blend into some abstract visionary setting which transforms their visible sign value into allusions. These allusions are, by virtue of the abstractions that enfold the objects, fully metaphoric. There is, of course, a rigorous unity in all of these works which coherently organizes the real and the imagined. The treatment of space in these paintings is multidirectional and establishes unstable relations among the elements, thus leading at times to an emotional claustrophobia and a modernist-postmodernist kind of tension. Furthermore, the spaces of these paintings move from the closed to the open and from the tightly framed to the loose and undefined.

"O body swayed
to music,
O brightening
glance,
How can we
know the
dancer
from the
dance?"

William Butler
Yeats

Music and Form

Emanuel's **"Orchestration," "Concerto"** and **"Ledger Line"** series are significant in a number of ways. First, the works are, because of their profound concern with music, partly rooted in the traditions of romantic art and vision. Given also that Iranian art is deeply touched by Romanticism and themes of music and musical instruments, then these paintings may also represent, in some modest measure, an attribute of Iranian art in exile. The paintings of other Iranian artists working in the West, such as Yunessi, Sabzi, Hessam and Zarin, to name a few, also bear similar morphological attributes. It should also be mentioned that music as a motif of romantic and visionary energies is also quite popular with cultures or peoples that have been assimilated into the cold and measured realities of the technological western societies. For these cultures, the energies that music exudes allude to dreamscapes that reject material reality in favor of ideals which can only be expressed in terms of melodies and musical fantasies. Moreover, musical symbolism in the arts signifies the inadequacies of language and its failure to express deeper sentiments.

In eastern paintings, these melodies have defined the dynamics of release, illusion, yearning and triumph. In truth, eastern art and specifically Iranian art, allows for music to burst forth with powers that overwhelm the realities of the flesh and reach into the infinity of the imagined and unsubstantiated emotional spaces. They are, in the last analysis, melodramatic and theatrical statements, deriving their energies from contradictions and irresolutions that exist between reality and dreams. These images which are amplified in the East are the sweet music of which the splendors are made. At the heart of their musical themes is a sense of remorse for the puritan dreams unfulfilled.

They all have a sense of inwardness and an internal dialogue about irreconcilable perspectives. The discourse that is generated from music alludes to romantic feelings for the infinite and evokes thoughts about the strangeness of the palpable and the beauty of the lost worlds and visions.

In transcendent cultures, whether they are religious or romantic, music as the most abstract of the arts is the voice of man's soul and addresses that which knowledge cannot ascertain. Music exists where language is a deficient sign for the understanding of the mysteries of being and of the world. The Surrealists and the Romantics found music to be the only means of expressing that which language was incapable of processing. For the Moderns, music became a symbol of the mysteries of subjective perceptions and a sign of the artist's unique expression. It allowed liberation from the monotony and the drudgery of everyday reality. In Persian art, it symbolizes the ultimate release of the soul into the transcendent spaces of love and of visions that only imagination can access. The more abstract it becomes, the more open-ended is its signification.

Persian art in exile is obsessed with musical symbolism and allusions. In these paintings music is the sign of love and piety, transcendence and heavenly visions. The **"Melodium"** series shifts the context from some golden gothic space to a more banal and everyday setting. Thus, it attributes to these features a sense of meaning that is metaphorically tangible. In **"Melodium"** the instruments establish myriad references to the objects of a world, and thus evoke a soul-image, that is fundamentally banal and everyday in its existence. If in the **"Concerto"** series the space widens into the ineffable, here the space

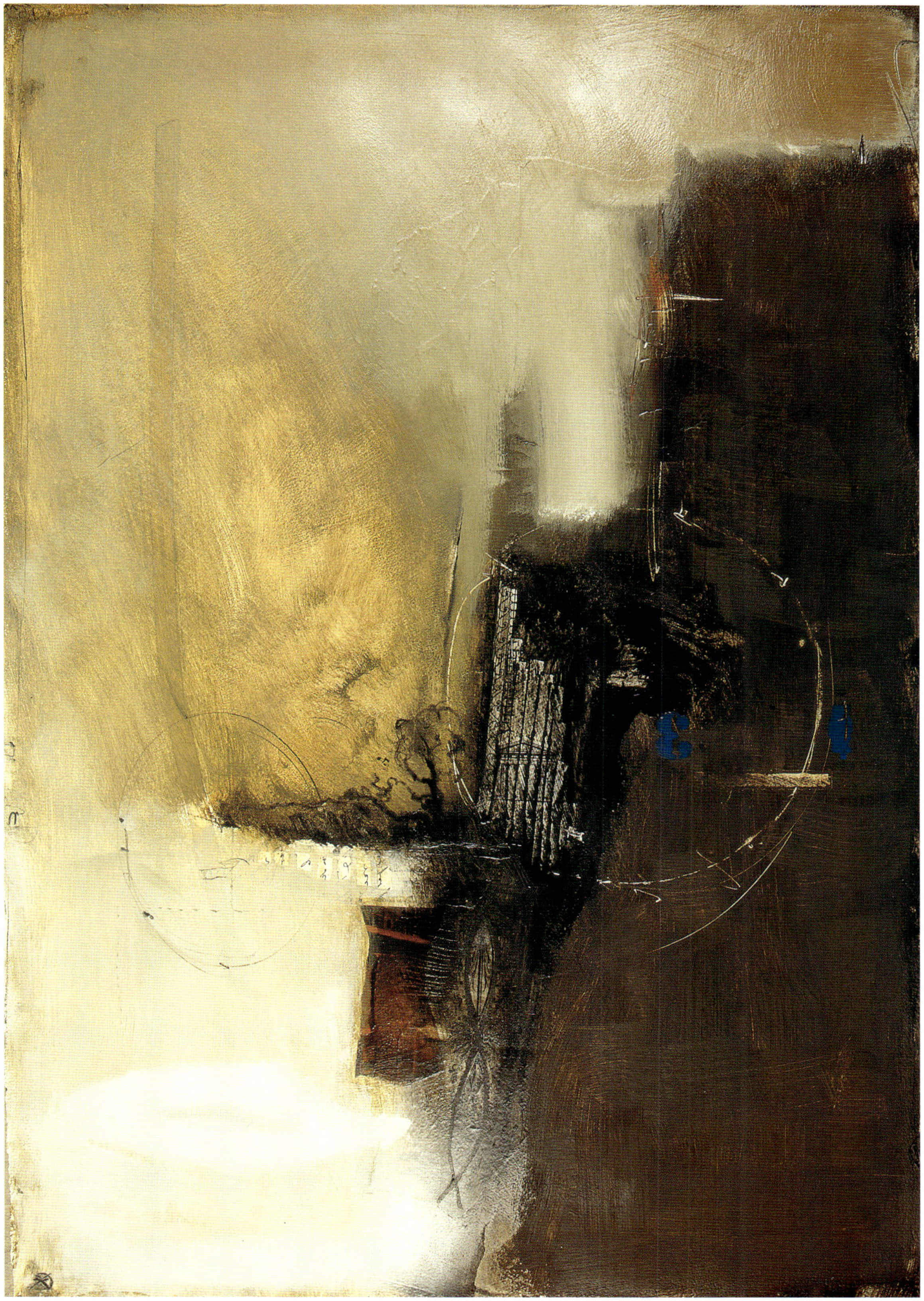

Hyperbole I

Mixed Media on Paper 30"x44"

narrows into the mundane. I must, however, add that the musical imagery in the works of other Iranian artists in exile, such as Hessam and Sabzi, often give in to conceit and a sensuousness that is ornate and even turgid. In Emanuel's paintings, however, his musical imagery does not have the theatricality and pathos, or the romantic excesses usually found in the works by other Iranian artists abroad. Emanuel's images have a laconic and simple face, both individually and compositionally. In fact, his designs, rather than his themes and their underlying spirit, associate the works more with the Moderns than the Romantics. The tone of his musical compositions is one of subjective expressions with a measured eye on the polemics of design rather than the disturbed and romantic emotional expressions.

These paintings establish a modernist vision of transforming all objective manifestations into abstract sensations. In other words, they evoke a sense of the world, more in terms of psychological release, than of material manifestations. The paintings address the essence of experience, reaching deeply into a subjective and solipsistic vision of being. This issue was a fascination of the European Orphists and the American Synchronists at the turn of the twentieth century and extending into the 1950s. The Orphists, however, such as Delaunay and Kupka, were more seriously devoted to art as music. One of these Orphists, the American Synchronist Stanton MacDonald Wright, went as far as attempting to correlate color and notation.

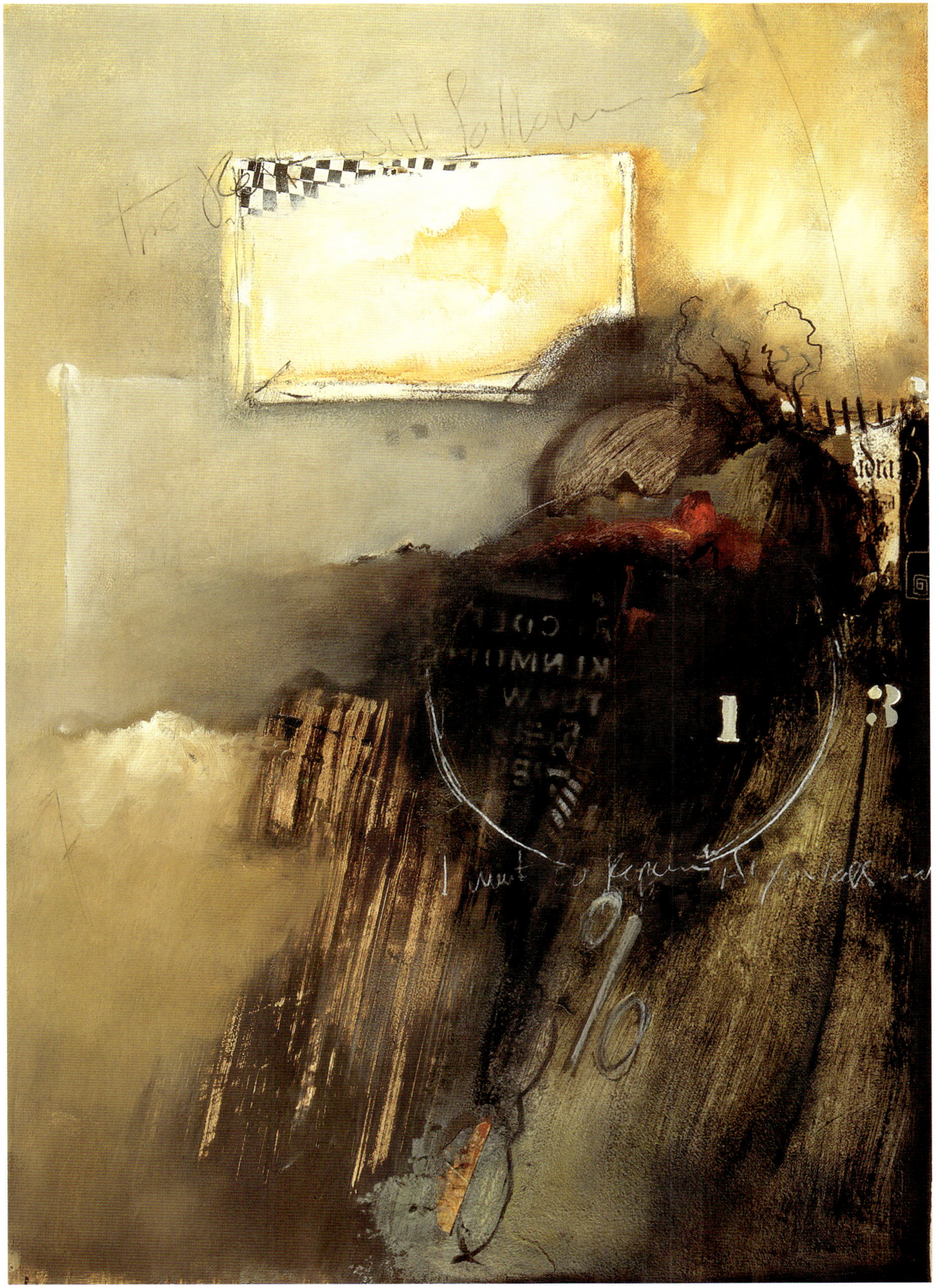

Hyperbole II

Mixed Media on Paper 30"x44"

In Emanuel's musical paintings, however, images are semiotically grounded—which distinctly separates him from the European or American Orphists. In Emanuel's works, it is the sign rather than the sensation resulting from its operation that is emphasized. In each painting, the signs stand for their linguistic signifiers. In other words, their meanings exist through the association of form and language. My point here is that the forms stand for their universals and thus establish transcendental ideologies regarding the images. In this regard the semiological aspect of the paintings grounds us in philosophical perspectives even though these views may not be cohesively ordered. Language thus remains as the defining force of the experience. For Emanuel, this issue stands in contra-distinction to the Orphists or the Synchronists, for the Orphists related to music as a sensational issue and not a semiological or linguistic one. Their aim was to give reign to sensations and obliterate the object or the image in the process. Emanuel's works, on the other hand, give priority to the image and thus assert its signifier-signified relationships. This point is crucial as the semiological dimension of Emanuel's paintings are a pre-eminent aspect of Postmodernism, alluding to the perseverance of language and the material quality of the world.

Index to Artwork

Index of Artwork

Abbas Daneshvari, Ph.D.

Art Historian and Critic, Abbas Daneshvari, Ph.D., has authored numerous articles, books and monographs on ancient, classic and modern art and architecture, specializing in western and middle eastern cultures. Professor of Art History at California State University, Los Angeles, Dr. Daneshvari holds degrees from UCLA, University of Massachusetts, Amherst and California State University, Hayward. His most recent book addresses contemporary, modern and postmodern art.

Book Design: Pamela Joy Trow-Johnson
Text: Abbas Daneshvari, Ph.D.
Editors: Christina Kline and Conal Byrne
Production Manager: Mehron Ebrahim Zadeh
Photography: Pezhman Deljou
Publisher: Deljou Art Group, Inc.

Emanuel: Vigil of a Winter's Moon
First Edition

Library of Congress Cataloging-in-Publication Data
ISBN: 0-9704356-0-6

Inquiries should be addressed to:
Deljou Art Group, Inc.,
1630 Huber Street, Atlanta, GA 30318
www.deljouartgroup.com

Printed in Singapore